Total Health

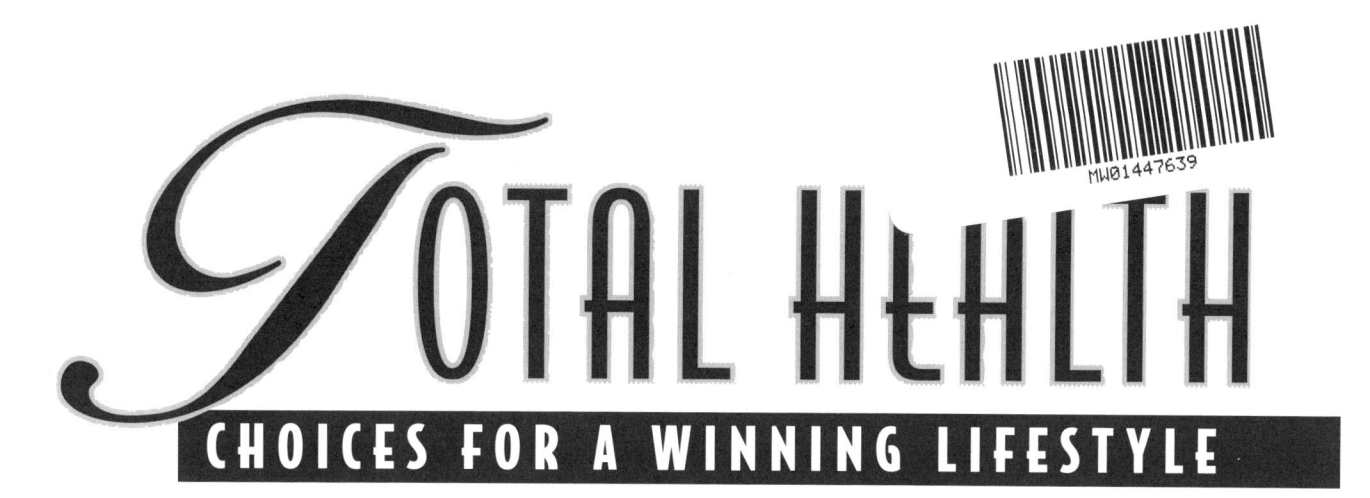

Choices for a Winning Lifestyle

Test and Quiz Master Book

SUSAN BOE

purposeful design
publications
A Division of ACSI

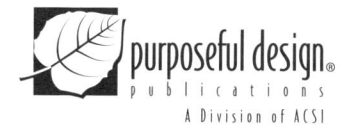

Colorado Springs, Colorado

Originally published 2000
© 2005 by ACSI/Purposeful Design Publications

All rights reserved. No portion of this book may be reproduced, stored in a retrieval system, or transmitted, in any form or by any means—mechanical, photocopying, recording, or otherwise—without prior written permission of ACSI/Purposeful Design Publications.

Purposeful Design Publications is the publishing division of the Association of Christian Schools International (ACSI) and is committed to the ministry of Christian school education, to enable Christian educators and schools worldwide to effectively prepare students for life. As the publisher of textbooks, trade books, and other educational resources within ACSI, Purposeful Design Publications strives to produce biblically sound materials that reflect Christian scholarship and stewardship and that address the identified needs of Christian schools around the world.

Printed in the United States of America
16 15 14 13 12 11 10 09 08 07   3 4 5 6 7

Boe, Susan
   Choices for a winning lifestyle: Test and quiz master book
   Second edition
   Total Health series
   ISBN 978-1-58331-228-5   Catalog #7609

Purposeful Design Publications
A Division of ACSI
PO Box 65130 • Colorado Springs, CO 80962-5130
Customer Service: 800-367-0798 • Website: www.acsi.org

Evaluation of Student Learning

Testing is only one way of evaluating a student's understanding and mastery of the material you are teaching. TOTAL HEALTH curriculum includes worksheets, vocabulary exercises, class discussions, group and individual projects from which to choose.

As a convenience, TOTAL HEALTH supplies one or two quizzes and one chapter test for each chapter. Based upon your class needs and teaching emphasis, these tests are designed as guides from which you can use all or part of each test. A unit test is not provided in the test and quiz book due to the fact that the teacher will write a unit test based upon the results of the quizzes and tests.

Although testing is often very stressful for students, it should not be a means to threaten or place undue stress upon students. Teachers must prepare students for evaluation. By no means does this mean to inform the students of the questions and answers. It does mean however, that the teacher should establish the testing based on what was taught, not on what is assumed known.

Each quiz and test supplied in the Total Health curriculum is designed to accommodate different learning styles:

- True and False
- Matching
- Short answer
- Essay: Note: if your students do not know how to write an essay, give them a brief discussion concerning the components of an essay. Do not grade too harshly on the format but more on the content, grammar, spelling, puncuation, and depth of understanding. If the students know what you expect, they are more likely to succeed.

The standard tests and quizzes supplied are neither too easy or too hard. Remember, these evaluations were written based on the textbook material, not on how the material was taught. Make your own adjustments to be sure you are testing the students fairly.

Copyright © 1995 Susan Boe

GRADING THE TESTS AND QUIZZES

The tests and quizzes combine both objective material (lists and information presented directly from the text), and subjective material (what the student gains from a Scripture, or what insight he has gained from a subject).

Each question is given a point value. I would suggest adding points as you grade the exams, looking for the positive rather than subtracting points, looking for the negative. Place a (+) beside each question rather than a (–). Then add up the points and come up with a (+) number at the top of the page. Divide this number by the total points available in the test and get a percentage. Use your school's percentage chart to arrive at a letter grade.

To save time and to give the students quick feedback, you can choose to correct the quizzes in class. Have the students pass the papers to a student or pass them into you and you pass them out again. The student correcting the quiz places his name at the top of the paper. Make sure you give instructions as to how you want the papers marked. Give the correct answers twice. If the student correcting a test has any questions concerning the quiz, a question mark should be placed next to the question number. The point value is placed at the top of the paper and then returned to the owner. Do not allow confrontation concerning the quiz results at this time. Tell the students you will go over them yourself and give the appropriate grade.

Ideas to use (in addition to tests and quizzes) for evaluation of student's learning:

- Explain questions from each chapter as daily assignments.
- Discussion questions from each chapter. Use as a writing assignment.
- Worksheets from each chapter.
- Vocabulary exercise(s) from each chapter.
- Suggested Activities from each chapter. Have the students do Key Concepts outline for each chapter as a regular assignment.
- Use the discussion questions at the end of each chapter for a speech or oral report.
- Use the suggested reading list from the Teacher's Edition for the students to complete a book report for each quarter.
- Use the TOTAL HEALTH Notebook for a quarter or semester project (see TOTAL HEALTH Notebook project from Teacher's Edition).
- Use the student's journal writing assignment(s) as a quarter or semester project.
- Use the discussion questions from each chapter as graded group discussions. Give each student a grade based on the evaluation provided in the Teacher's Edition.
- Use the students' teaching from chapter 2 Systems of the Body as described in the Teacher's Edition as a graded project.

GRADING ESSAYS AND SHORT ANSWER QUESTIONS

Many students find it difficult to communicate what they know through writing. You can help your students develop this skill by incorporating writing in health class. The standard tests given in the TOTAL HEALTH curriculum provide an essay question. In most cases the essay question is objective with points written next to the proper information to be included in the essay. There are times, however, where the question may be more subjective. You need to evaluate the answer based on some concrete issues such as grammar, punctuation, spelling and completeness of answer. You need to teach the students how you want your essay questions answered and then give them the practice they need to develop a positive attitude toward writing and a successful experience in test taking. Note the following example:

Essay: 25 points: Teenagers generally have poor eating habits. They are also prone to developing eating disorders such as anorexia, bulimia, or chronic overeating. Write an essay called:

"Teens and their eating habits"

Include in your essay:
1. Why teens typically have poor eating habits.
2. Why it is important for teens to eat well.
3. Suggestions for healthy snacks.
4. Signs of anorexia or bulimia.
5. What you might say to a friend who shows signs of an eating disorder.

It is logical from the questions that each may be worth 5 points to add up to 25 points. Each question may carry a different amount of weight based on the depth of the required response. Use your own judgment with the point values based on how you taught the class.

If the students only list the answers, they have not written an essay but a list. Explain how to develop an opening statement. Help them with transition from point to point and a good conclusion.

The following is a sample answer based upon points #1 and #2 in the above essay to illustrate one essay grading style:

+ Good opening statement   +5 Good points!

Generally teens have poor eating habits. These eating habits are caused by the following factors: hurried lifestyle, lack of discipline, variety of food choices, the feeling of being indestructible, and lack of knowledge. It is important for teens to eat well because their bodies are growing rapidly and maturing through puberty. Furthermore, teens are developing lifestyle habits. Good nutrition is needed for academic success and energy is needed for physical activity.

+5

Point values can vary depending upon what concepts were emphasized when the material was taught.

TOTAL HEALTH — CHAPTER 1: QUIZ

Unit 1: Physical Health

KEY

Sections: 1-1, 1-2, 1-3
25 points

DEFINE: (1 point each) Define the following terms as they are defined in the text.

1. Anatomy: *Anatomy is the field of study dealing with the structure of body parts, their forms and arrangements.*
2. Physiology: *Physiology is the field of study dealing with the function of body parts, what they do and how they do it.*
3. Homeostasis: *Homeostasis is the condition of a stable internal environment.*
4. Cells: *Cells are the basic building blocks from which all larger parts are formed.*
5. Tissues: *Tissues are made up of similar cells that are specialized to carry on particular functions in the body.*

SHORT ANSWER: (2 points each) Answer the following questions.

6. What is the goal of all body structures and functions?
    The goal of all body structures and functions is to maintain life.

7. What system of the body is the only system that has a separate function from the total human body, and what is its function?
    The reproductive system is the system that has a separate function from the total human body. Its primary function is to reproduce.

8. Explain the unique relationship between the organs in your body and the systems in your body.
    The body is like a team. Each one of its members needs to be functioning the way it was designed so the whole body can accomplish its task. Every organ of your body needs to be healthy and functioning to ensure the health of the eleven systems of your body.

9. List the five factors that the human body depends upon for survival. (5 points)
   1. Water
   2. Food
   3. Oxygen
   4. Heat
   5. Pressure

10. **ESSAY:** Explain what is meant by the following scripture. How might this affect the way you live? Matthew 6:25,32–35. (9 points)

   "Therefore I say to you, do not worry about your life, what you will eat or what you will drink; nor about your body, what you will put on. Is not life more than food and the body more than clothing?…For your heavenly Father knows that you need all these things. but seek first the kingdom of God and His righteousness, and all these things shall be added to you." Matthew 6:25, 32–35

   Possible Answer: The scripture in Matthew 6 means that God knows all my needs, physical, mental, social and spiritual. If I worry about my life I am not trusting the Lord to take good care of me. If I can learn to trust God with every area of my life, it would change the way I live. My priorities change from trying to meet my own needs to thinking more about the needs of others, like my friends and family. If I seek what God wants for my life and not so much about what I want for my life, God will take care of me.

TOTAL HEALTH — CHAPTER 1: TEST

Unit 1: Physical Health

KEY

100 points

DEFINE (2 points each): Use complete sentences and define the following terms as they are defined in the text.

1. Organs: *Two or more tissues grouped together and performing specialized functions.*
2. Systems of the body: *Related organs make up the systems of the body.*
3. Cells: *The basic building blocks from which all larger parts are formed.*
4. Homeostasis: *The condition of a stable internal environment.*
5. Tissues: *Are made up of similar cells that are specialized to carry on particular functions in the body.*

6. Why did Jesus have such a special place in His heart for children? How are we to come to Christ? (5 points)

    A child's faith and gratitude is simple and uncomplicated. We are to come to Christ as children.

7. Why are anatomy and physiology often discussed together? (5 points)

    They are closely related. It is difficult to separate the structure of body parts from their function.

8. Why is homeostasis so important in the human body? Give one example. (5 points)

    The body has a constant need to maintain balance. When the environment outside the body changes, temperature or oxygen for example, the conditions within the body must remain stable.

9. The body's internal thermostat is set at 98.6°F. Explain how homeostasis relates to the body's need to maintain this temperature? How does the body accomplish this? (5 points)

    If the temperature drops, the body automatically triggers the brain to generate heat, and the body may begin to shiver. If the body is too hot, the brain may turn on the body's natural cooling system and the body begins to sweat.

Copyright © 1995 Susan Boe

Chapter One, Test Key, page 2 of 3

10. Explain the unique relationship between the organs in your body and the systems in your body. (5 points)

    The body is like a team. Every organ in the body needs to be healthy and functioning to ensure the health of the 11 systems of the body.

11. Who invented the microscope? Why did this invention change the course of scientific research? (4 points)

    Anton Van Leeuwenhoek. He opened the doors to the invisible world. Researchers use the microscope as the basis for scientific development.

12. What is meant by the following phrase: "My body, composed of many parts, is one." (5 points)

    The body works together to function as one healthy being. Many smaller parts, such as the cells and tissues form larger parts that eventually make up the whole body, as one complete being.

13. List the eleven systems of the body. (1 point each)
    1. *Circulatory*
    2. *Respiratory*
    3. *Skeletal*
    4. *Muscular*
    5. *Digestive*
    6. *Excretory*
    7. *Integumentary (skin)*
    8. *Endocrine*
    9. *Nervous*
    10. *Immune*
    11. *Reproductive*

MATCHING (2 points): For each item on the left column, find an appropriate answer on the right column. Place the letter of the correct answer in the space provided at the left of each item. Each answer can be used only once.

14. _C_ Epithelial tissue
15. _E_ Muscle tissue
16. _D_ Connective tissue
17. _A_ Organs
18. _F_ Nerve tissue

A. Two or more tissues grouped together and performing specialized functions.
B. Related organs.
C. Sheets that cover all body surfaces, inside and out.
D. Tendons, ligaments, bone and cartilage.
E. Cause body parts to move.
F. Receive and transmit impulses to various parts of the brain.

TRUE-FALSE (2 points each): If the answer is true, put a T to the left of the item number. If the answer is false, put an F to the left of the item number. Please respond to each item.

T 19. The primary function of the muscle tissue is to contract.
T 20. Epithelial tissues can reproduce quickly in case cells are damaged or injured.
F 21. Skeletal muscles are called involuntary muscles.
T 22. The skin is an organ.
T 23. The entire human body is made up of cells.

24. **ESSAY** (25 points): Write an essay (more than two paragraphs) to respond to the following question. Check for proper spelling and punctuation.

What does the following scripture mean to you? How might this affect the way you live?

"For Thou didst form my inward parts; Thou didst weave me in my mother's womb. I will give thanks to Thee, for I am fearfully and wonderfully made; Wonderful are Thy works, and my soul knows it very well." Psalm 139:13-14

Possible Answer: God has made me very special. There is no one else like me and He knows every part of my being inside and out. It is awesome when I think about how magnificent God made the human body. If I really believe in my heart that God made me and that I am special, then I know that no matter how I look His love for me is great because He made me this way! God does not make mistakes!

Psalm 139 can positively affect the way I live. My self esteem is tied into the wrong things that the world would like me to believe is important. (include in paragraph portions from chart page 3 in student text). I know that God loves me and He wants me to develop things in my life that the world may not think are important -- but He does and that's what really counts!

TOTAL HEALTH

CHAPTER 2: QUIZ A

Unit 1: Physical Health

KEY

Sections: 2-1, 2-2, 2-3
25 points

DEFINE: (1 point each) Use complete sentences and define the following terms as they are defined in the text.

1. Circulatory system: *The circulatory system is the group of body parts that transports the blood throughout the body to keep the body functioning properly.*
2. Arteriosclerosis: *Arteriosclerosis is a disease where certain arteries become hardened and obstructed, eventually limiting or stopping the flow of blood to certain organs of the body.*
3. Respiratory system: *The respiratory system is the group of passages that exchanges gases in order for the body to function properly.*
4. Bronchitis: *Bronchitis is a swelling or inflammation of the bronchi.*
5. Skeletal system: *The skeletal system is the combination of the joints and connecting tissues.*

MATCHING (1 point each): For each item on the left column, find the appropriate answer on the right column. Place the letter of the correct answer in the space provided at the left of each item. Each answer can be used only once.

6. _D_ Arthritis:
7. _F_ Muscular system:
8. _A_ Digestive system:
9. _B_ Ulcer:
10. _E_ Excretory system:

A. The organs that take in food and break it down into a chemical form that can be absorbed by the body.
B. Studies indicate that this condition is caused by a bacteria.
C. A conditioned caused when the formation of bile in the gallbladder forms into crystals.
D. The inflammation of a joint or joints.
E. Includes the large intestine as the main organ.
F. The group of tissues that makes the body parts move.

Copyright © 1995 Susan Boe

SHORT ANSWER: Answer the following questions (2 points each).

11. What are the two jobs of the kidneys?

    These organs function as the cleansers of the blood as well as regulators of the body's fluid content.

12. How can a person give him or herself a blood transfusion? Why might someone consider doing this procedure?

    Blood transfusions can pass on diseases from the person who donates the blood to the person receiving the blood. A person can give himself a blood transfusion by donating his own blood ahead of time for use when the operation takes place.

13. Explain the meaning of the terms inspiration and expiration.

    Inspiration means to inhale air into the alveoli where the oxygen in the air passes through the alveoli into the veins that carry it to the heart. During expiration or exhalation, carbon dioxide (a waste product) is carried up the airways and out of the body.

14. Explain how the skeletal system is like the framework for your body.

    The bones are like a framework for the body because they provide support and protection. The bones hold the body upright and when you lie down to sleep they still provide support for the organs and muscles.

15. Explain the following principle as it relates to the muscles in the body: "With every action, there is an equal and opposite reaction." Include one example in your answer.

    Muscles work in pairs. With every movement of a muscle there is another muscle working as well. For example, when bringing a basketball into proper shooting position, your biceps muscle is shortened but your triceps muscle is lengthened. As you shoot the ball, your biceps muscle is lengthened and the triceps muscle is shortened.

16. **ESSAY** (5 points): In essay form respond to the following situation:
    A good friend of yours has begun to smoke cigarettes. You have decided to confront him and encourage him to stop. Include a minimum of five reasons for him to stop the habit.
    - Cost
    - Cancer
    - Addictive
    - Makes clothes smell bad
    - Not "cool" any more

TOTAL HEALTH

CHAPTER 2: QUIZ B

Unit 1: Physical Health

KEY

Sections: 2-4, 2-5
25 points

DEFINE: (1 point each) Use complete sentences and define the following terms as they are defined in the text.

1. Integumentary system: *The integumentary system is the system of the body which includes the skin, hair, nails, sweat glands and oil glands.*
2. Natural immunity: *Natural immunity is the body's resistance to certain diseases.*
3. Acquired immunity: *Acquired immunity occurs when the body adapts to respond to certain invaders and then can remember who the intruders were so next time they are ready to attack.*
4. Central nervous system: *The central nervous system controls and coordinates all the body parts so that they work as one flowing unit and respond to changes appropriately.*
5. Endocrine system: *The glands of the endocrine system secrete hormones to send messages to the cells in the body by way of the blood.*

MATCHING (1 point each): For each item on the left column, find the appropriate answer on the right column. Place the letter of the correct answer in the space provided at the left of each item. Each answer can be used only once.

6. _C_ Immune system
7. _F_ Diabetes
8. _A_ HIV
9. _E_ Autoimmune disease
10. _B_ Epilepsy

A. The virus that causes AIDS.
B. A brain disorder that results from a sudden burst of nerve action.
C. The group of organs and cells that works with the lymphatic system to fight germs.
D. A disease in which the outer coating that protects some nerves is destroyed.
E. A condition when the body's immune system mistakes its own cells and tissues for possible intruders.
F. A disease where the body cannot properly utilize the glucose (sugar) that it needs.

TRUE OR FALSE: (1 point each) If the answer is true, put a T to the left of the item number. If the answer is false, put an F to the left of the item number. Please respond to each item.

_T_ 11. The fingerprints of identical twins are not exactly alike.
_F_ 12. Warts on the skin are caused by a bacteria.
_T_ 13. Immunodeficiency disorders result in the body's failure to fight infection.
_F_ 14. Cerebral Palsy is a condition resulting from a spinal injury.

SHORT ANSWER (2 points each): Answer the following questions.

15. Explain the functions of the hormones in your body.
    - *Energy control*
    - *Sugar and insulin balance*
    - *Water and salt balance*
    - *Growth and sexual maturity*
    - *Menstruation cycle in females*
    - *Affect emotions such as anger, fear, joy and sadness*

16. What are two possible results of prolonged exposure to the sun?
    - *Increase risk of skin cancer*
    - *Accelerates aging process*

17. What are two symptoms a person may experience when their immune system is not functioning effectively?
    - *Repeat bouts with colds or flu viruses*
    - *Continual fatigue*
    - *Increased allergic reactions*
    - *Incomplete recovery from a sickness*
    - *Poor response to treatment when sick*

18. **ESSAY** (5 points): The endocrine system works closely with the nervous system and it affects the reproductive system. Explain the function of the endocrine system, include in your essay the following points:
    - The function of the endocrine system.
    - How is the nervous system and endocrine system different?
    - What are "chemical messengers? Give 3 of their functions?
    - How does the endocrine system affect the reproductive system?

    Answer: The essay should clearly explain the above points:
    - *The endocrine system is responsible for maintaining an internal balance in the body. It accomplishes this by secreting hormones.*
    - *The nervous system and endocrine system both maintain an internal balance in your body. However, the glands of the endocrine system secrete hormones to send messages to the cells in the body by way of the blood.*
    - *These hormones are called "chemical messengers." They have many functions. Hormones are responsible for a child's growth over a period of time, they are responsible for regulating a female's menstruation cycle and they also affect a person's emotions.*
    - *The endocrine system affects the reproductive system directly by the release of hormones that cause the maturing of the male and female reproductive organs.*

TOTAL HEALTH — CHAPTER 2: TEST

Unit 1: Physical Health

KEY

100 points

DEFINE (2 points each): Use complete sentences and define the following terms as they are defined in the text.

1. Circulatory system: *The circulatory system is the group of body parts that transports the blood throughout the body to keep the body functioning properly.*
2. Arteriosclerosis: *Arteriosclerosis is a disease where certain arteries become hardened and obstructed, eventually limiting or stopping the flow of blood to certain organs of the body.*
3. Bronchitis: *Bronchitis is a swelling or inflammation of the bronchi.*
4. Natural immunity: *Natural immunity is the body's resistance to certain diseases.*
5. Endocrine system: *The group of body parts that uses chemicals (hormones) secreted by the glands to send messages to the cells in the body by way of the blood.*

TRUE OR FALSE (2 points each): If the answer is true, put a T to the left of the item number. If the answer is false, put an F to the left of the item number. Please respond to each item.

- _F_ 6. The integumentary system is the system responsible for transporting the blood throughout the body.
- _T_ 7. Arteries carry oxygenated blood away from the heart.
- _T_ 8. Anemia is a condition characterized by a shortage of red blood cells.
- _T_ 9. A person's lifestyle can influence hypertension.
- _F_ 10. The female reproductive system includes the ovaries, the uterus and the testes.

Chapter Two, Test Key, page 2 of 4

MATCHING (2 points each): For each item on the left column, find the appropriate answer on the right column. Place the letter of the correct answer in the space provided at the left of each item. Each answer can be used only once.

11. _D_ Veriform appendix
12. _F_ Food poisoning
13. _A_ Tonsils
14. _C_ Alimentary canal
15. _E_ Ulcer

A. Often a source of infection.
B. Expels waste in the form of urine.
C. Measures about 30 feet in length.
D. A pouchlike structure that contains lymphatic tissue.
E. An open sore in the lining of the stomach.
F. May cause damage to your liver and may cause death.

SHORT ANSWER: Answer the following questions.

16. You can help avoid food poisoning by following 4 guidelines, what are they? (4 points)
    1. *Do not eat food from cans that are dented or are bulging.*
    2. *Do not eat foods that have not been kept refrigerated or stored properly.*
    3. *Do not eat any food that has an unusual discoloration or odor.*
    4. *Do not eat foods that have not been cooked thoroughly such as poultry, beef and pork.*

17. Explain the following principle as it relates to the muscles in your body; "with every action, there is an equal and opposite reaction." Include one example in your answer. (5 points).
    With every movement of a muscle there is another muscle working. For example, consider the movement of shooting a basketball. As you bring the ball into proper position, your biceps muscle is shortened but your triceps muscle is lengthened. As you shoot the ball, your biceps muscle is lengthened and your triceps muscle is shortened.
    Other examples: legs: quadriceps and hamstrings
    back: back muscles and stomach muscles

18. What are two possible results of prolonged exposure to the sun? (2 points)
    1. *Increase chance of skin cancer*
    2. *Accelerated aging process*

19. The skin has several important functions, list and explain 3 functions of the skin. (6 points)
    1. *Protection: from water and infection*
    2. *Regulation of body temperature: protects internal organs and body temperature from extreme cold and heat.*
    3. *Sensitivity: Sensory receptors on the skin enable you to feel sensations of pressure, touch, heat, cold and pain.*

20. What is diabetes? Include in your answer its relationship with the hormone insulin and what can be done to control the disease. (3 points)
    Diabetes is an example of a disease where the body cannot properly utilize the glucose (sugar) that it needs. This disorder has to do with the release and use of the hormone insulin. A careful diet or insulin shots might be needed to control this condition.

21. **ESSAY** (25 points): The name of this chapter is *Eleven Systems: One Body*. Explain what is meant by the fact that all your eleven systems form one body. You will receive 5 points for including each of the following in your answer.
    1. The name of each of the eleven systems of the body.
    2. How each of the eleven systems interacts with other systems.
    3. The primary function of each system.
    4. One problem for each system and what can be done for that problem.

Possible Answer:

- *Circulatory, respiratory, skeletal, muscular, digestive, excretory, integumentary, immune, nervous, endocrine and reproductive systems.*

- *The respiratory system exchanges gases that the circulatory needs to transport throughout the body by way of the veins and arteries. The skeletal and muscular system use the oxygen that the respiratory and circulatory system brought in. They also protect the organs of the systems and give the body stability. The muscles give the bones a way of movement. The digestive system breaks down foods and the excretory system gets rid of the waste from the food and the other waste produced by the body. The skin gives all the systems a form of protection and covering. The immune system works to fight off diseases that could cause each system to malfunction. The endocrine works with each system to help balance the body's internal environment. The reproductive system is the only system that is independent from most of the other systems other than the endocrine system.*

- *Main functions of each system:*
  Circulatory: transports blood throughout the body (four main functions pg. 27).
  Respiratory: group of passages that exchanges gases.
  Muscular: provides movement.
  Skeletal: provides a framework for the body.
  Digestive: break down food into chemical form for absorption.
  Excretory: provides ways for wastes to be expelled from the body.
  Integumentary: provides protection, sensitivity, and regulation of body temperature.
  Nervous: maintains a stable internal environment.
  Endocrine: secretes hormones to send messages to the cells in the body via the blood.
  Reproductive: to produce offspring.

- *Problem for each and what can be done for that problem (see appropriate sections for each system in student text).*

22. **ESSAY** (25 points): It is important to show respect toward others. How can teens show respect for another's privacy in the area of sexuality? Include in your answer:
    - Why are people often uneasy discussing the reproductive systems?
    - How is your knowledge of your reproductive system closely related to your perspective on your sexuality?
    - How can teens specifically show respect to one another?
    - How does God view the human body?

Possible answer:
- *Natural inborn modesty. God-given to help us respect each other's privacy.*
- *God made man and woman special and unique in every way. The reproductive system functions the way God designed it to function, with a purpose. It helps you feel secure in knowing God made you this way for a reason. And to keep His purposes as a motivation to keep yourself sexually pure.*
- *Not talking or asking personal questions to other teens, not joking about the body or sexual feelings or attitudes. Not asking anyone to do something that would be against God's best for that person.*
- *God views the human body, both male and female, as beautiful. He was not ashamed to create male and female and we should not be ashamed of our bodies either.*

TOTAL HEALTH

CHAPTER 3: QUIZ A

Unit 1: Physical Health

KEY

Sections: 3-1, 3-2
25 points

DEFINE (1 point each): Define the following terms as they are defined in the text.

1. Protein: *Nutrients needed by the body for building new tissue.*
2. Carbohydrates: *Energy producing foods such as starches and sugars.*
3. Cholesterol: *A waxy substance that is carried around the body in the bloodstream by lipoproteins.*
4. Basal Metabolism: *The ability of the body to use energy at a higher rate when the body is at rest.*
5. Calorie: *A unit of heat the body uses for energy.*

MATCHING (1 point each): For each item on the left column, find the appropriate answer on the right column. Place the letter of the correct answer in the space provided at the left of each item. Each answer can be used only once.

6. _D_ LDL
7. _B_ HDL
8. _E_ Complex carbohydrates
9. _F_ Amino acids
10. _C_ Saturated fat

A. Does not tend to increase cholesterol levels.
B. Good cholesterol.
C. Tends to increase cholesterol levels.
D. Bad cholesterol.
E. Starches that are broken down by the body into two or more sugars.
F. The chief component of every protein.

SHORT ANSWER: Answer the following questions (note the points given to each question).

11. List the six main kinds of nutrients that the body needs. (6 points)

    1. *Proteins*
    2. *Carbohydrates*
    3. *Fats*
    4. *Vitamins*
    5. *Minerals*
    6. *Water*

Copyright © 1995 Susan Boe

Chapter Three, Quiz A Key, page 2 of 2

12. Give two reasons it can be very difficult to make wise food choices? (2 points)
    - *Many unhealthy food choices available.*
    - *Researchers are continually finding new information concerning healthy food choices.*
    - *The increased role of the fast food industry.*

13. Give two of the six reasons why fats are an essential part of the diet. (2 points)
    - *Growth and repair*
    - *Maintaining body temperature*
    - *Cushioning of vital organs*
    - *Insulation of the body through the stored fat in tissues*
    - *Keeping the skin from becoming dry and flaky*
    - *Manufacture of certain hormones*

14. **ESSAY** (5 points):
    If God were to write you a prescription for good nutrition what would it include? Name and explain the ten statements of the prescription for good nutrition.
    1. *Eat a variety of foods*
    2. *Maintain ideal weight*
    3. *Use exercise to keep your metabolism high*
    4. *Increase dietary fiber to 25–35 grams a day*
    5. *Eat less sugar*
    6. *Eat less sodium*
    7. *Eat less fat*
    8. *Avoid alcohol and smoking*
    9. *Drink plenty of water*
    10. *Avoid eating while under stress*

TOTAL HEALTH — CHAPTER 3: QUIZ B

Unit 1: Physical Health

KEY

Sections: 3-3, 3-4
25 points

DEFINE (1 point each): Define the following terms as they are defined in the text.

1. Vitamins: *Organic substances the body needs to help regulate and coordinate functions of the body.*
2. Minerals: *Minerals are inorganic substances essential for your body to help form bones, teeth and blood cells.*
3. Set Point Theory: *The theory that a body maintains a certain comfort zone, a weight that is difficult to break.*
4. Anorexia: *Anorexia is self-induced starvation resulting in extreme weight loss and characterized by an intense fear of gaining weight and becoming fat.*
5. Bulimia: *Bulimia is a pattern of bingeing (eating large amounts of food) followed by self-induced vomiting or laxative abuse with or without weight loss.*

FILL-IN THE BLANK: Fill-in the appropriate answer for the following (note the points given to each question).

6. _Recommended Daily Allowance_ or RDA is a broad-based percentage to help guide you in your dietary choices. (1 point)
7. You may see a label marked _fortified_ with essential vitamins. This means that the product has added vitamins above what it would have had naturally. (1 point)
8. You may see a label marked _enriched._ This means that vitamins and minerals were added to the product after some of the nutrients were removed during processing. (1 point).
9. "If you do not take time for _health_ today, you will have to take time for _sickness_ tomorrow." (2 points)
10. A mystery term often listed on products is _"hydrogenated"_ oil. This is a chemical process used to make unsaturated fat more saturated. (1 point)

Copyright © 1995 Susan Boe

11. List the four sources of calories and include the calories per gram that each contain. (8 points)

Source	Calories per gram
1. Carbohydrates	4
2. Protein	4
3. Fat	9
4. Alcohol	7

12. **ESSAY** (6 points): Reading labels is a three-step process. Explain each step and include an example for each.
    1. *Do not be swayed by packaging: for example "lite" or "light."*
    2. *See if the actual amount of fat and cholesterol are listed. For example, hold two boxes of cereal next to each other and compare the serving size with each ingredient listed.*
    3. *Be aware of the types of oils contained in the product. For example, "one or more of the following" coconut oil and safflower oil. You cannot make an educated choice. It is wise, however, to avoid all tropical oils.*

TOTAL HEALTH

CHAPTER 3: TEST

Unit 1: Physical Health

KEY

100 points

DEFINE (2 points each): Define the following terms as they are defined in the text.

1. Complex carbohydrates: *Starches that are broken down by the body into two or more sugars.*
2. Cholesterol: *A waxy substance that is carried around the body in the bloodstream by lipoproteins.*
3. Basal Metabolism: *The ability of the body to use energy at a higher rate when the body is at rest.*
4. Glucose: *The result of the break down of carbohydrates into a type of sugar that provides fuel for the body.*
5. Insulin: *A hormone released from the pancreas to regulate the sugar in the body.*

TRUE OR FALSE (2 points each): If the answer is true, put a T to the left of the item number. If the answer is false, put an F to the left of the item number.

- _F_ 6. One gram of fat contains 4 calories.
- _T_ 7. It takes 3,500 stored calories to make one pound of fat.
- _F_ 8. Vitamin supplements are a good replacement when you are not eating right.
- _F_ 9. Fat-soluble vitamins are those that can be excreted from the body.
- _T_ 10. Chronic overeating is far more common than anorexia or bulimia.

FILL-IN BLANK AND SHORT ANSWER:

11. The principle of weight loss is _calories_ in _calories_ out. (2 points)
12. Today's healthy eating plan stresses _what_ you eat, rather than _how much_ you eat, and stresses an _active_ lifestyle rather than a _sedentary_ one. (4 points)
13. What is the role of fiber in the diet? (1 point)
    It is not a nutrient but acts like a broom through the intestines and carries with it unwanted waste.

Chapter Three, Test Key, page 2 of 3

14. List three of the five keys to keeping an effective food journal. (5 points)
    1. *Be totally honest with yourself. Write down everything.*
    2. *Be as exact as possible.*
    3. *Make no dietary changes when you begin your journal.*
    4. *Write down the time of day you eat or drink something.*
    5. *Be accountable to someone.*

15. List the 6 main kinds of nutrients. (6 points)
    1. *Proteins*   4. *Vitamins*
    2. *Carbohydrates* 5. *Minerals*
    3. *Fats*   6. *Water*

16. Carbohydrates are *energy*   *producers*   for the body. (1 point)

17. Explain the difference between LDL cholesterol and HDL cholesterol. (4 points)
    LDL is low density lipoproteins (the bad cholesterol). LDL tends to be deposited in the arteries. HDL is high density lipoproteins (good cholesterol). HDL is removed from circulation and transported to the liver to be eliminated.

18. Fill in the following Food Guide Pyramid with the correct food groups. Include the amount of servings suggested for each group. (12 points).

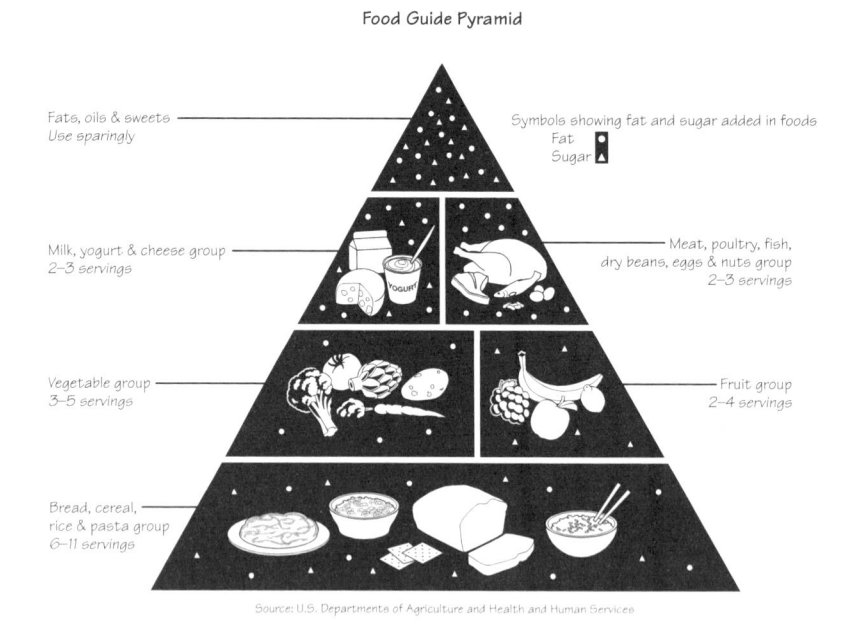

Food Guide Pyramid

- Fats, oils & sweets — Use sparingly
- Symbols showing fat and sugar added in foods
  - Fat
  - Sugar
- Milk, yogurt & cheese group — 2–3 servings
- Meat, poultry, fish, dry beans, eggs & nuts group — 2–3 servings
- Vegetable group — 3–5 servings
- Fruit group — 2–4 servings
- Bread, cereal, rice & pasta group — 6–11 servings

Source: U.S. Departments of Agriculture and Health and Human Services

19. **ESSAY** (20 points): List and explain each item on the *Prescription of Good Nutrition* from the chapter. (1 point for listing and 1 point for explaining each)
    1. *Eat a variety of foods.*
    2. *Maintain ideal weight.*
    3. *Use exercise to keep your metabolism high.*
    4. *Increase dietary fiber to 25-35 grams a day.*
    5. *Eat less sugar.*
    6. *Eat less sodium.*
    7. *Eat less fat.*
    8. *Avoid alcohol and smoking.*
    9. *Drink plenty of water.*
    10. *Avoid eating while under stress.*

20. **ESSAY** (25 points): Teenagers generally have poor eating habits. They are also prone to developing eating disorders such as anorexia, bulimia, or chronic overeating. Write an essay called:

    "Teens and their eating habits."

    Include in your essay:
    1. Why teens typically have poor eating habits.
    2. Why it is important for teens to eat well.
    3. Suggestions for healthy snacks.
    4. Signs of anorexia or bulimia.
    5. What you might say to a friend who shows signs of an eating disorder.

    1. *Teens have poor eating habits because of schedule and lack of knowledge*
    2. *Teens are growing especially during puberty and need good nutrition for the physical and emotional changes.*
    3. *Healthy snacks: fruit, vegetables, etc.*
    4. *Signs of anorexia or bulimia include: change in eating patterns, extreme weight loss.*
    5. *Do not try to counsel them or tell them to eat. Tell them you care and you want them to talk to their parents or get counsel.*

TOTAL HEALTH — CHAPTER 4: QUIZ A

Unit 1: Physical Health

KEY

Sections: 4-1, 4-2, 4-3
25 points

DEFINE (1 point each): Define the following terms as they are defined in the text.

1. Fitness: *The ability of the whole body to work together to the highest level possible.*
2. Blood pressure: *The measure of the resistance to blood flow in the vessels and the efficiency of circulation.*
3. Lean body weight: *The weight of muscles in the body.*
4. Aerobic: *When the body demands more oxygen than normal.*
5. Anaerobic: *Short bursts of energy, without the use of oxygen.*

MATCHING (1 point each): For each item on the left column, find the appropriate answer on the right column. Place the letter of the correct answer in the space provided at the left of each item. Each answer can be used only once.

6. _B_ Overload
7. _D_ Progression
8. _A_ Specificity
9. _F_ Cross training
10. _C_ Lifetime sports

A. You must do certain exercises to develop different body parts.
B. Gradually do more than normal to improve performance.
C. Those activities that you can continue as you get older.
D. Starting with a little and adding to it regularly as you improve.
E. The volume of blood pumped by the heart in one minute.
F. Putting a variety in your exercise routine.

Chapter Four, Quiz A Key, page 2 of 2

SHORT ANSWER: Answer the following questions (note the points given to each question).

11. List the four parts to physical fitness. (4 points)
    1. *Cardiovascular fitness*
    2. *Muscular fitness*
    3. *Flexibility*
    4. *The body's fat-vs-lean relationship*

12. Explain why exercise is good for the heart muscle. (3 points)
    1. *Resting heart rate and the rate at which your heart beats during exercise will decrease.*
    2. *Cardiac output will improve (the volume of blood pumped by the heart in one minute).*
    3. *Stroke volume will improve (the volume of blood the heart pumps at each stroke).*
    4. *Helps control your blood pressure.*
    5. *Helps your heart resist the number one killer, cardiovascular disease.*

13. What is the number one killer in America? (1 point)
    Cardiovascular disease or heart disease

14. Give two reasons why exercise is so important in weight control. (2 points)
    1. *Exercise increases your metabolism so that calories are burned not only during exercise but for hours afterward.*
    2. *Regular exercise increases your lean muscle mass and muscle burns more calories than fat.*
    3. *Your body will look toned and fit.*

15. ESSAY (5 points)
    Explain why the following statement is a false statement:

    "I have to be good at sports to be involved in exercise."

    Being involved in sports does not guarantee you are fit. Furthermore, a personal exercise program is just that, personal. It is designed with you in mind to create a program that best suits your strengths and weaknesses. Although you do not need skill in a specific sport to be involved in exercise, being skilled at some activity may increase your enjoyment of that activity.

TOTAL HEALTH

CHAPTER 4: QUIZ B

Unit 1: Physical Health

KEY

Sections: 4-4, 4-5, 4-6
25 points

DEFINE (1 point each): Define the following terms as they are defined in the text.

1. Atrophy: *A condition when a muscle is not used and it decreases in size and loses its strength.*
2. Target heart rate: *A way to monitor the intensity of a workout, so the heart and lungs can benefit the most from a workout.*
3. Insomnia: *The inability to go to sleep.*

SHORT ANSWER: Answer the following questions (note the points given to each question).

4. Explain what realistic goals are and give three of the six goals you might consider when setting exercise goals. (4 points)
    Realistic goals are goals that you set that fit you personally. For example, muscular strength, weight loss or weight gain, inches lost or gained, competition, overall physical well-being, or improvement in specific health related problem or injury.

5. List the six components that every exercise program should include. (6 points)
    1. *Type of activity: "What should I do?"*
    2. *Intensity: "How hard should I work?"*
    3. *Duration: "How long should I work out?"*
    4. *Frequency: "How often should I work out?"*
    5. *Maintenance: "How long should I keep up my program?"*
    6. *Motivation: "How can I stay motivated?"*

6. Explain the following diagram and how it relates to monitoring your level of intensity during a workout. (2 points)

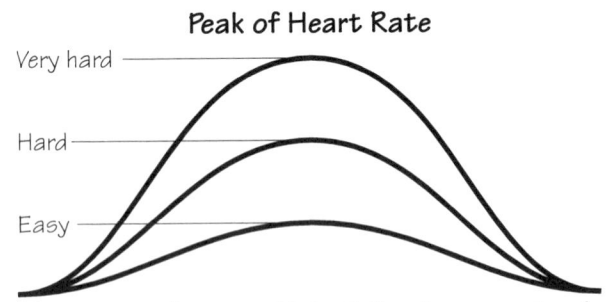

Peak of Heart Rate
Very hard
Hard
Easy

While you are working out it is important to monitor your level of intensity. You should periodically check your pulse throughout your workout to measure it against your target heart rate. After you have been exercising on a consistent basis, you may be able to ask yourself the following question based on the chart. "How hard am I working?" You may experience this progression several times during one workout session and your intensity may change with how you are feeling on that particular day. To reach a comfortable level during your workout, you must alternate periods of higher intensity with periods of lower intensity.

7. List 5 of the 10 ideas to keep you motivated to keep up an exercise program. (5 points)
    1. *Keep an exercise journal.*
    2. *Make and evaluate your goals continually.*
    3. *Plan a regular program and follow it.*
    4. *Add music or speaking tapes to your workout.*
    5. *Enter a competition or fun walk/run.*
    6. *Train with a friend.*
    7. *Join a club or group or take lessons.*
    8. *Be accountable to someone.*
    9. *Reward yourself when you have reached a goal.*
    10. *Add fun activities to your program (bike, hike, trip etc.).*

8. List the 3 types of fatigue. (3 points)
    1. *Physical fatigue.*
    2. *Emotional fatigue.*
    3. *Fatigue due to illness.*

9. Sleep seems to be one of the first things teenagers go without. Give two reasons why it is important for you to get enough sleep. (2 points)
    - *Improves ability to concentrate.*
    - *Your body is changing and growing and needs sleep.*
    - *Improves the amount of energy you have.*
    - *Improves your ability to cope with life.*
    - *Improves your overall attitude about life.*

21. What is the purpose of knowing your target heart rate? Show the formula you would use to figure your own target heart rate. To receive full points you must show what your personal target heart rate is. (10 points)

22. **ESSAY** (25 Points): You are to write out a personal exercise program for yourself. Include in your program the following:
    1. Your realistic fitness goals you want to accomplish. (5 points)
    2. The six components that every exercise program should include. (6 points)
    3. How you will monitor your heart and intensity during a workout. (5 points)
    4. Five ideas you will use to help keep you motivated. (5 points)
    5. What you will do if you get injured. Use the acronym RICE. (4 points)

23. **ESSAY** (25 points): Sleep is a necessary part of your physical existence. Sleep is the time when the body can restore itself. Write an essay entitled:

    "Teens and their sleep habits"

    Include in your essay the following:
    1. Why teens typically have poor sleeping habits. (5 points)
    2. The five stages of sleep that are necessary for a good night's sleep. (5 points)
    3. Five hints for a better night's sleep. (5 points)
    4. Matthew 11: 28-30 "Come to Me all you who labor and are heavy laden, and I will give you rest...." Explain what it means to "rest in God." (5 points)
    5. How you can improve your own personal sleep habits. (5 points)

TOTAL HEALTH

CHAPTER 4: TEST

Unit 1: Physical Health

KEY

100 points

DEFINE (2 points each): Define the following terms as they are defined in the text.

1. Fitness: *The ability of the whole body to work together to the highest level possible.*
2. Blood pressure: *The measure of the resistance to blood flow in the vessels and the efficiency of circulation.*
3. Lean body weight: *The weight of the muscles in the body.*
4. Atrophy: *A condition when a muscle is not used and it decreases in size and loses its strength.*
5. Insomnia: *The inability to go to sleep.*

TRUE OR FALSE (2 points each): If the answer is true, put a T to the left of the item number. If the answer is false, put an F to the left of the item number.

__F__ 6. Exercise will make you hungry.
__F__ 7. Weight training will make you have large, bulky muscles.
__T__ 8. An Ergogenic Aid is something that improves physical work performance.
__T__ 9. Pressing against the wall is an example of Isometric exercise.
__T__ 10. Isokinetic exercise is a combination of isometric and isotonic exercise.

FILL-IN THE BLANK AND SHORT ANSWER:

11. The most important measurement of your fitness is __cardiovascular__ fitness. (2 points)
12. A __contraction__ is a shortening or pulling of the muscle that causes movement to occur. (2 points)
13. Muscles are made up of two fibers, __fast twitch__ and __slow twitch__ fibers. (2 points)
14. An __EKG or (electrocardiogram)__ records the electrical impulses set off by the heart. (2 points)
15. __Realistic__ goals are goals that you set for yourself personally. (2 points)

Copyright © 1995 Susan Boe

16. What made Covert Bailey change his view of exercise? (2 points)

    He went running with a friend and he could not go very far without stopping and vomiting. He realized that running put his friend in shape to play squash but that squash failed to put him in shape for running. He then developed an interest in steady, uninterrupted exercise known as aerobics.

17. Explain the following diagram and how it relates to monitoring your level of intensity during a workout. (5 points)

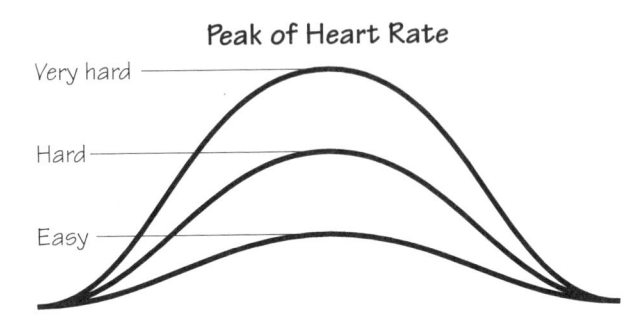

    Peak of Heart Rate
    Very hard
    Hard
    Easy

    While you are working out it is important to monitor your level of intensity. You should periodically check your pulse throughout your workout to measure it against your target heart rate. After you have been exercising on a consistent basis, you may be able to ask yourself the following question based on the chart. "How hard am I working?" You may experience this progression several times during one workout session and your intensity may change with how you are feeling on that particular day. To reach a comfortable level during your workout, you must alternate periods of higher intensity with periods of lower intensity.

18. List the four parts to physical fitness. (4 points)
    1. *Cardiovascular fitness*
    2. *Muscular fitness*
    3. *Flexibility*
    4. *The body's fat-vs-lean relationship*

19. Give two reasons why exercise is so important in weight control. (2 points)
    1. *Exercise increases your metabolism so that calories are burned not only during exercise but for hours afterward.*
    2. *Regular exercise increases your lean muscle mass and muscle burns more calories than fat.*
    3. *Your body will look tone and fit.*

20. Sleep seems to be one of the first things teenagers go without. Give two reasons why it is important for you to get adequate sleep. (2 points)
    - *Improves ability to concentrate.*
    - *Your body is changing and growing and needs sleep.*
    - *Improves the amount of energy you have.*
    - *Improves your ability to cope with life.*
    - *Improves your overall attitude about life.*

21. What is the purpose of knowing your target heart rate? Show the formula you would use to figure your own target heart rate. To receive full points you must show what your personal target heart rate is. (10 points)

    (5 points) Target heart rate gives you a range at which you should monitor your intensity during a workout. It is good to know so you can get the most benefit out of a workout.

    (3 points) Formula for figuring target heart rate:
    220 – age = maximum heart rate or danger zone
    80% of the maximum = higher limit
    60% of the maximum = lower limit

    (2 points) for figuring their own (see textbook page 110)

22. ESSAY (25 Points): You are to write out a personal exercise program for yourself. Include in your program the following:
    1. Your realistic fitness goals you want to accomplish. (5 points)
    2. The six components that every exercise program should include. (6 points)
    3. How you will monitor your heart and intensity during a workout. (5 points)
    4. Five ideas you will use to help keep you motivated. (5 points)
    5. What you will do if you get injured. Use the acronym RICE. (4 points)

    Answer:
    1. *Personal.*
    2. *Type of activity, intensity, duration, frequency, maintenance, motivation.*
    3. *Target heart rate and/or hard, easy, chart.*
    4. *Music, do it with a friend, join a club, keep a journal, use an exercise video.*
    5. *Rest the injured area. Ice the area. Compress. Elevate.*

23. **ESSAY** (25 points): Sleep is a necessary part of your physical existence. Sleep is the time when the body can restore itself. Write an essay entitled:

"Teens and their sleep habits"

Include in your essay the following:
1. Why teens typically have poor sleeping habits. (5 points)
2. The five stages of sleep that are necessary for a good night's sleep. (5 points)
3. Five hints for a better night's sleep. (5 points)
4. Matthew 11: 28-30 "Come to Me all you who labor and are heavy laden, and I will give you rest...." Explain what it means to "rest in God." (5 points)
5. How you can improve your own personal sleep habits. (5 points)

Answer:
1. *Schedule, discipline, time management.*
2. *Stage 1, 2, 3, 4 and REM.*
3. *Wind down, get regular exercise, eat a balanced diet, get up earlier, have a consistent bed time, avoid eating right before bed, avoid alcohol and caffeine, give your cares and worries to God, avoid sleeping aids, avoid heavy exercise before bed.*
4. *Personal, subjective.*
5. *Personal, subjective.*

Chapter Five, Quiz A Key, page 1 of 2

TOTAL HEALTH

CHAPTER 5: QUIZ A

Unit 1: Physical Health

KEY

Sections: 5-1, 5-2, 5-3
25 points

DEFINE (1 point each): Define the following terms as they are defined in the text.

1. Disease: *Any condition that negatively affects the normal functioning of the mind or body.*
2. Infectious disease: *All diseases that are caused by the spread of germs.*
3. Pathogens: *Germs or microorganisms that cause disease.*
4. Acute disease: *Those diseases that develop suddenly with symptoms that are often severe.*
5. Chronic disease: *Diseases that develop gradually and may persist for years.*

MATCHING (1 point each): For each item on the left column, find the appropriate answer on the right column. Place the letter of the correct answer in the space provided at the left of each item. Each answer can be used only once.

6. __C__ Bacteria
7. __D__ Virus
8. __D__ Fungi
9. __F__ Allergen
10. __B__ Antibodies

A. Your ability to fight the invading germ.
B. Special proteins produced by the lymphocytes.
C. One-celled tiny organisms that come in many shapes and grow everywhere.
D. Organisms that usually cause diseases of the skin.
E. Responsible for more infections than any other pathogen.
F. A substance to which your body is particularly sensitive to.

Copyright © 1995 Susan Boe

Chapter Five, Quiz A Key, page 2 of 2

FILL-IN THE BLANK AND SHORT ANSWER: Answer the following questions (note the points given to each question).

11. Label the following diagram: (4 points)

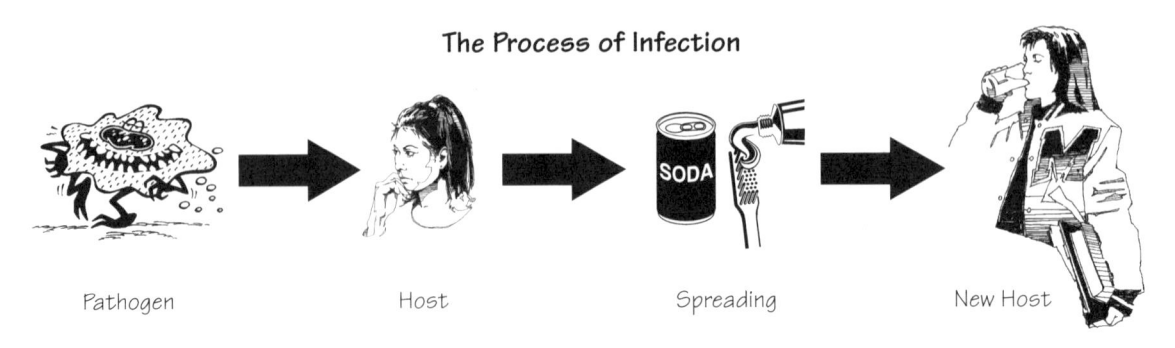

The Process of Infection

Pathogen → Host → Spreading → New Host

12. The _incubation period (or contagious period)_ is the most infectious time of the disease but is usually hard to pinpoint because it is usually during the early stages of the disease. (1 point)

13. List the three ways that germs can be spread and give an example for each. (6 points)
    1. *Direct contact*   *example: Sexually transmitted diseases*
    2. *Contact with objects*   *example: Sharing drinking glasses*
    3. *Contact with animals*   *example: Bites from various insects*

14. **ESSAY** (4 points): God designed the human body with its own physical armor to battle the war against sickness. Explain the body's physical defenses. To receive full credit you must give four ways your body was created to protect you from sickness.
    - *Your skin*
    - *Mucous membrane*
    - *Hair on the skin, in the nose and ears*
    - *Blinking of the eyes*
    - *Eyelashes*
    - *Vomiting*
    - *Diarrhea*
    - *Antibodies*

TOTAL HEALTH — CHAPTER 5: QUIZ B

Unit 1: Physical Health

KEY

Sections: 5-4, 5-5
25 points

MATCHING (1 point each): For each item on the left column, find the appropriate answer on the right column. Place the letter of the correct answer in the space provided at the left of each item. Each answer many be used only once.

1. _C_ Chlamydia:
2. _E_ Gonorrhea:
3. _A_ Sterility:
4. _D_ Syphilis:
5. _B_ Herpes Simplex II:

A. Incapable of producing offspring.
B. The STD that causes painful sores on the genital area.
C. The most common of the sexually transmitted diseases yet the most difficult to discover.
D. Often called the "great imitator" because it looks like so many other STD's.
E. Often called the "preventer of life" because it can cause sterility in both males and females.
F. Causes cold sores or blisters on or around the mouth.

TRUE OR FALSE (1 point each): If the answer is true, put a T to the left of the item number. If the answer is false, put an F to the left of the item number.

_T_ 6. When you take medication for a cold, you are not treating the virus but only the symptoms of the virus.
_F_ 7. Mononucleosis results in a high number of red blood cells in the body.
_F_ 8. Hepatitis A is much more serious than Hepatitis B.
_T_ 9. A form of pneumonia is an opportunistic infection.
_T_ 10. The AIDS virus attacks a person's immune system.

Copyright © 1995 Susan Boe

Chapter Five, Quiz B Key, page 2 of 2

SHORT ANSWER: Answer the following questions (note the points given to each question).

11. Why have scientists been unable to find a cure for the common cold? (1 point)
    Because scientists have found that the cold virus is caused by many different viruses.

12. List four of the five suggestions for fighting the common cold. (4 points)
    1. Eat well
    2. Get plenty of rest
    3. Exercise regularly
    4. Keep the stress in your life in balance
    5. Avoid smoking

13. **ESSAY** (5 points): Write an essay entitled:
    "The physical consequences of becoming sexually active."

    Answer:
    STD's (they should list the diseases)
    PID for females (Pelvic Inflammatory Disease)
    Sterility
    AIDS, HIV

TOTAL HEALTH   CHAPTER 5: TEST

Unit 1: Physical Health

KEY

100 points

DEFINE (2 points each): Define the following terms as they are defined in the text.

1. Disease: *any condition that negatively affects the normal functioning of the mind or body.*
2. Infectious disease: *All diseases that are caused by the spread of germs.*
3. Pathogens: *Germs or microorganisms that cause disease.*
4. Acute disease: *Those diseases that develop suddenly with symptoms that are often severe.*
5. Chronic disease: *Diseases that develop gradually and may persist for years.*

TRUE OR FALSE (2 points each): If the answer is true, put a T to the left of the item number. If the item is false, put an F to the left of the item number.

 _F_ 6. Gonorrhea is the most common of the sexually transmitted diseases yet the most difficult to discover.
 _T_ 7. Syphilis is often called the "great imitator" because it looks like so many other STD's.
 _F_ 8. Chlamydia is often called the "preventor of life" because it can cause sterility in both males and females.
 _F_ 9. Herpes Simplex I causes painful sores on the genital area.
 _T_ 10. Sterility is the inability to produce offspring.

FILL IN THE BLANK AND SHORT ANSWER:

11. _Mononucleosis_ is a viral infection that results in a high number of white blood cells in the blood. (2 points)
12. _Viruses_ are responsible for more infections than any other pathogen. (2 points)
13. Scientists have found that a _vaccine_, a mixture of weakened or killed germ cells, will cause the body to produce enough _antibodies_ for that particular disease. (4 points)
14. The only true _safe sex_ is _no sex_. (2 points)

Copyright © 1995 Susan Boe

15. Explain the role of the lymphatic network in the defense against disease. (4 points)
    The second line of defense after your skin. Lymph nodes manufacture white blood cells called lymphocytes which travel through the lymphatic network fighting off germs.

16. Explain the function of the T-cells and B-cells in the lymphatic network. (2 points)
    The two kinds of lymphocytes are called the T-cells and B-cells. These white blood cells and antibodies act like warriors for your body by destroying individual germ cells and help the body organize an attack against groups of germs cells.

17. Scientists have discovered that the AIDS virus destroys T-cells. How might this affect the body's immune system? (5 points)
    Since T-cells help the B-cells as well as specifically fight the disease. They also make a mental picture of the attacking disease so if it tries to enter again, the body is prepared to fight it. If the T-cells are destroyed, the body cannot effectively fight off diseases.

18. List four of the five suggestions for fighting the common cold. (4 points)
    1. *Eat well*
    2. *Get plenty of sleep*
    3. *Exercise regularly*
    4. *Keep the stress in your life in balance*
    5. *Avoid smoking*

19. What are the physical consequences of becoming sexually active? (5 points)
    STD's
    Sterility
    AIDS
    HIV
    Pelvic Inflammatory Disease

20. **ESSAY** (25 points): Thoroughly describe the infectious disease process.
    Answer: The pathogen (germ), the host, how it can be spread, and the new host. The answer should be thorough.

21. **ESSAY** (25 points): The body has physical defenses against sickness, but we are also equipped with spiritual defenses. What are these spiritual defenses and how can a person find peace even in the midst of an illness.

Answer: Spiritual defenses:
> *Prayer, the Word of God, Keep an attitude of Faith.*
> *God is with those who are sick, and He gives grace to handle difficult situations. The answer should be more thorough.*

TOTAL HEALTH — CHAPTER 6: QUIZ A

Unit 1: Physical Health

KEY

Section: 6-1
25 points

DEFINE (1 point each): Define the following terms as they are defined in the text.

1. Degeneration: *A lowering of effective power, vitality, or essential quality to a worsened kind or state; to pass from a higher to a lower type or condition.*
2. Noninfectious Disease: *(noncommunicable): Diseases caused by heredity, the environment, and a person's lifestyle and are not passed on from one person to another.*
3. Degenerative Disease: *The body's tissues break down and do not grow or function properly.*
4. Genetic Disorder: *A disease or condition caused primarily by a defect or defects in the inherited, genetic material within a person's genes.*
5. Congenital: *Genetic disorders that are evident at birth.*

MATCHING (1 point each): For each item on the left column, find the appropriate answer on the right column. Place the letter of the correct answer in the space provided at the left of each item. Each answer can be used only once.

6. _C_ Regenerate
7. _E_ Birth Defects
8. _D_ Lifestyle diseases
9. _A_ Risk factors

A. Traits or habits that raise someone's chances of getting a disease.
B. A lowering of effective power.
C. To restore or renew.
D. Caused by your health habits.
E. Abnormalities obvious at birth or detectable early in infancy.

FILL-IN THE BLANK AND SHORT ANSWER: Answer the following questions (note the points given to each question).

10. _Prevention_ is very important in fighting degenerative diseases. (1 point)
11. As the result of _sin_ Adam and Eve's relationship with God changed as did their _mental_ and _physical_ conditions. (3 points)

Copyright © 1995 Susan Boe

12. For as by one man's _disobedience_ many were made sinners, so also by one Man's _obedience_ many will be made righteous. (2 points)
13. Explain the meaning of the phrase: "God is sovereign and full of grace." (2 points)
    God has all power and authority and is completely in control of everything. He is full of grace, that is, He gives unmerited favor and love to His people.

14. List three physical hazards that may cause illness. (3 points)
    1. *Air pollution.*
    2. *Water pollution.*
    3. *Solid waste pollution.*

15. **ESSAY** (5 points): Lifestyle diseases may start developing at an early age. Explain how teenagers can make positive lifestyle choices to help in the prevention of noninfectious diseases. Include in your answer specific examples of positive lifestyle choices.

    Answer should include the following plus specific examples teens can make.
    - *Balanced and nutritious diet.*
    - *Sleep.*
    - *Exercise.*
    - *Dealing with stress.*
    - *Avoiding tobacco, alcohol, drugs.*

Chapter Six, Quiz B Key, page 1 of 2

TOTAL HEALTH

CHAPTER 6: QUIZ B

Unit 1: Physical Health

KEY

Section: 6-2
25 points

MATCHING (1 point each): For each item on the left column, find the appropriate answer on the right column. Place the letter of the correct answer in the space provided at the left of each item. Each answer may be used only once.

1. _D_ Arteriosclerosis
2. _E_ Hypertension
3. _A_ Cancer
4. _F_ Carcinogens
5. _B_ Benign

A. A condition caused by abnormal cells growing without control.
B. The description of a non-cancerous tumor.
C. The description of a cancerous tumor.
D. Hardening of the arteries.
E. High blood pressure.
F. The substances around you that cause cancer.

TRUE OR FALSE (1 point each): If the answer is true, put a T to the left of the item number. If the answer is false, put an F to the left of the item number.

_T_ 6. Atherosclerosis is the buildup of fat deposits on the artery wall.
_F_ 7. A stroke may result when damage to part of the heart has been caused by a blockage of blood supply or leakage of blood outside the artery wall.
_F_ 8. A tumor that is called a malignant tumor is not cancerous in nature.
_T_ 9. Diabetes mellitus results when the pancreas does not produce adequate amounts of insulin.
_F_ 10. Hypoglycemia is an abnormally high level of sugar in the blood.
_T_ 11. Multiple sclerosis is a progressive disease of the central nervous system.
_F_ 12. Muscular dystrophy is the most common acquired disease in young adults.

Copyright © 1995 Susan Boe

SHORT ANSWER: Answer the following questions (note the points given to each question).

13. Why is high blood pressure often called the "silent killer"? (1 point)
    High blood pressure is often called the silent killer because there are no outward signs of the disease until it is too late.

14. According to the American Cancer Society, what is the meaning of the acronym **CAUTION**? (7 points)
    Change in bowel or bladder habits
    A sore that does not heal
    Unusual bleeding or discharge
    Thickening or lump in the breast or elsewhere
    Indigestion or difficulty swallowing
    Obvious change in a wart or mole
    Nagging cough or hoarseness

15. **ESSAY** (5 points): A person's diet, scientists say, may have much to do with an individual's susceptibility to cancer. What can you do in the fight against cancer? Include in your answer 4 dietary habits a person should adopt in the fight against cancer and include one personal dietary change you could make to help your diet fight against cancer.

    - *Eat a diet rich in fruits (especially rich in vitamin C), vegetables and fiber, and low in fat.*
    - *Eat vegetables rich in beta carotene (broccoli, cantaloupe, carrots, spinach, squash).*
    - *Eat a diet rich in calcium (low-fat dairy products).*
    - *Eat fewer salty and highly processed foods.*
    - *Personal dietary change*

TOTAL HEALTH — CHAPTER 6: TEST

Unit 1: Physical Health

KEY

100 points

DEFINE (2 points each): Define the following terms as they are defined in the text.

1. Noninfectious Disease: *(noncommunicable): Disease caused by heredity, the environment, and a person's lifestyle and are not contagious.*
2. Degenerative Disease: *The body's tissues break down and do not grow or function properly.*
3. Genetic disorder: *A disease or condition caused primarily by a defect or defects in the inherited, genetic material within a person's genes.*
4. Congenital: *Genetic disorders that are evident at birth.*
5. Lifestyle diseases: *Diseases caused by your health habits.*

TRUE OR FALSE (2 points each): If the answer is true, put a T to the left of the item number. If the item is false, put an F to the left of the item number.

_T_ 6. A stroke may result when damage to part of the brain has been caused by a blockage of blood supply or leakage of blood outside the artery wall.
_T_ 7. A tumor that is called benign is a non-cancerous tumor.
_F_ 8. Hypoglycemia is an abnormally high level of sugar in the blood.
_T_ 9. Arteriosclerosis is hardening of the arteries.
_F_ 10. Muscular dystrophy is the most common acquired disease in young adults.
_F_ 11. Metastasis is the name given to tumors that remain in one location in the body.
_T_ 12. A biopsy is a microscopic examination of tissue cells.

FILL IN THE BLANK AND SHORT ANSWER: Answer the following questions (note the points to each question).

13. The specific cause of cancer is not known. However, there are certain factors that researchers believe increase a person's chances of developing cancer. List the 5 factors that contribute to the development of cancer. (5 points)
    1. *A person's genetic makeup (inherited).*
    2. *Lifestyle habits.*
    3. *Environmental factors.*
    4. *Occupational hazards.*
    5. *Body's reaction to a virus.*

14. According to the American Cancer Society, what is the meaning of the acronym **CAUTION**? (7 points):
    *C**hange in bowel or bladder habits*
    *A** sore that does not heal*
    *U**nusual bleeding or discharge*
    *T**hickening or lump in the breast or elsewhere*
    *I**ndigestion or difficulty swallowing*
    *O**bvious change in a wart or mole*
    *N**agging cough or hoarseness*

15. _Prevention_ is very important in fighting degenerative diseases. (2 points)
16. Those people who suffer from diabetes type I are _insulin_ dependent. (2 points)
17. _Arthritis_ is characterized by pain, swelling, stiffness, and redness of the joints. (2 points)
18. Whatever the situation, _compassion_ for those who suffer from any noninfectious disease is important. (2 points)
19. One of the most important things you can do to help avoid certain diseases is to _know your medical history._ (2 points)
20. _Alzheimer's disease_ is a progressive condition in which nerve cells in the brain degenerate and the brain loses its ability to function. (2 points)
21. What is the primary concern of someone who has diabetes? (2 points)
    The primary concern of someone who has diabetes is to keep the blood sugar level in balance.

22. What is the meaning of the following verse? How can it relate to your physical *and* spiritual condition?

    "For as by one man's disobedience many were made sinners, so also by one Man's obedience many will be made righteous" (Romans 5:19). (5 points)

23. **ESSAY** (20 points): "An ounce of prevention is worth a pound of cure." This is certainly true when it comes to high blood pressure and heart disease. Write an essay explaining what teenagers can do to help them in the prevention of heart disease. Include in your answer:
    - Why is high blood pressure often called the "silent killer"?(2 points)
    - What are 5 factors that may lead to an increase risk of developing high blood pressure? (5 points)
    - What are the 4 risk factors that are out of your control concerning heart disease? (4 points)
    - What are the preventative measures against heart disease? (9 points)

    Answer:
    - *Silent killer because you cannot see symptoms until you have high blood pressure. You cannot feel high blood pressure.*
    - *5 factors: family history, obesity, tobacco smoking, eating large amounts of salt extreme stress, diabetes melitus.*
    - *Risk factors out of your control: family history, air, water and solid waste.*
    - *Preventative measures: Regular screening of blood pressure, reduce your weight, do not smoke, reduce or stop drinking alcohol, eat a healthy diet, exercise, learn to manage stress.*

24. **ESSAY** (25 points): Write an essay entitled:
"What I can do in my own personal fight against cancer."

Include in your answer: (5 points each)
- Why is prevention the best medicine?
- What dietary changes can you make to help fight cancer?
- What type of self-tests can I do to help detect cancer?
- What are the warning signs of cancer?
- What are the ways cancer is treated?

Possible Answer may include:
- *prevention is the best and most inexpensive way to prevent illness. You can keep your risk factors low if you help prevent disease by your lifestyle choices.*
- *Vitamin A, Vitamin C, eat plant-rich foods and natural antioxidants "clean-up" free radicals (cancer causing agents). see list page 167 in student text.*
- *CAUTION spells: Change in bowel or bladder habits. A sore that does not heal. Unusual bleeding or discharge. Thickening or lump in the breast or elsewhere. Indigestion or difficulty swallowing. Obvious change in wart or mole. Nagging cough or hoarseness.*
- *Surgery, Chemotherapy, Radiation (also natural means such as herbs and dietary changes have helped some).*

TOTAL HEALTH — CHAPTER 7: QUIZ A

Unit 2: Mental Health

KEY

Sections: 7-1, 7-2
25 points

DEFINE (1 point each): Define the following terms as they are defined in the text.

1. Stress: *The body's response to external or internal changes.*
2. Stressor: *The stimulus that triggers the stress.*
3. Positive stress: *Stress that challenges a person enough to face daily responsibilities and to pursue life goals.*
4. Distress: *Stress that reaches a point when feelings of depression, confusion and exhaustion replace the natural excitement and drive to meet a challenge.*

TRUE OR FALSE (1 point each): If the answer is true, put a T to the left of the item number. If the answer is false, put an F to the left of the item number.

_F_ 5. Type B personality is also known as "hurried sickness."
_T_ 6. The "fight or flight" response is a natural way of dealing with a stressful situation.
_T_ 7. When distress occurs, the results of the stress on your life can be fatal.
_F_ 8. There are increased health risks to a person who has a Type B personality.

FILL IN THE BLANK AND SHORT ANSWER: Answer the following questions (note the points given to each question).

9. An important key to understanding your mental health is the phrase, "how well do you respond to your _environment?"_ (1 point)
10. Happiness is a by-product of responding to life from _God's_ perspective. It is not determined by your _circumstances_ but by your _attitudes_ and responses to them. (3 points)

Copyright © 1995 Susan Boe

Chapter Seven, Quiz A Key, page 2 of 3

11. People respond differently to the same stressor. List 4 factors that affect a person's reaction to stress. (4 points)
    1. *The person's age, social status, income, cultural background, stage in life and previous experiences.*
    2. *The circumstances surrounding the situation.*
    3. *How much control the person has or thinks he/she has over the situation.*
    4. *The personality of the person. Type A or B?*
    5. *The person's personal relationship with God.*

12. Explain why it is important to have some stress in your life and give one example of why this is important. (2 points)
    A person needs some stress to challenge them to meet the responsibilities of each day. For example, if you did not have to get out of bed to go to school, you would not be motivated to get out of bed.

13. List 4 effects of negative stress (1 from each category). (4 points)
    PHYSICAL: *loss of appetite, high blood pressure, stroke, headache, anorexia nervosa, loss of menstruation, obesity, cancers of many types, mono, strep, asthma.*
    MENTAL: *Irritability, low self-esteem, depression, lack of creativity, more critical of others and self, grades suffer.*
    SOCIAL: *Uninvolved with friends, angry outbursts, poor time management, lack of communication.*
    SPIRITUAL: *Uninvolved in spiritual activities, no time to pray or read the Word, feelings of guilt and depression, dissatisfaction in life.*

14. **ESSAY** (3 points): A proper view of stressful situations is in Romans 8:28:

"And we know that God causes all things to work together for good to those who love God, to those who are called according to His purpose" (NAS).

Write an essay explaining how your faith in God and in His Word can make a difference in handling stress.

Possible Answer may include:
- *Each person's life has meaning.*
- *Faith in God and in His word can help to lighten the load and get the proper perspective concerning the circumstances.*
- *God is with you in your deepest trials.*
- *You are on the best team, God's team, and you are a very important part of that team.*
- *God works all things for good to those who love Him.*
- *Peace in your heart that surpasses understanding can help you in your circumstances.*

TOTAL HEALTH   CHAPTER 7: QUIZ B

Unit 2: Mental Health

KEY

Sections: 7-3. 7-4
25 points

FILL IN THE BLANK AND SHORT ANSWER: Answer the following questions (note the points given to each question).

1. No matter what your religious belief, the _Bible_ is a positive prescription for living a healthy life. (1 point)

2. List 5 ways to deal with stress. (5 points)

   1. *Eat well.*
   2. *Get plenty of sleep.*
   3. *Laugh if off.*
   4. *Talk things out with someone.*
   5. *Learn to relax.*
   6. *Learn to say "no" to extra activities.*
   7. *Set priorities.*
   8. *Don't let worry drain you.*
   9. *Learn not to procrastinate.*
   10. *Get moving!*
   11. *Time management.*
   12. *Exercise.*
   13. *Write it down: keep a journal.*

3. List 5 signs of depression. (5 points)

   1. *Inability to sleep.*
   2. *Decrease in appetite.*
   3. *Feeling bored and unmotivated.*
   4. *Losing interest in activities of life.*
   5. *Inability to concentrate.*
   6. *Feeling of fatigue.*

4. Explain why depression is like the "common cold" of mental disorders. (3 points)
   It starts with little sniffles; no one dies of the sniffles. But without proper care, a cold (or depression) can progress from the sniffles to a head cold, to a chest cold and even to pneumonia... plenty of people die of pneumonia. It is also very common and natural to feel depressed at times.

5. Our _attitude_ determines our _action._ (2 points)

6. Explain what it means to be a "tough-minded optimist" and how this type of attitude might affect the way you handle stress. (4 points)

A tough-minded optimist is a person who doesn't break apart in his thoughts whatever the stress and who continues hopefully and cheerfully to expect the good no matter what the apparent situation. This is having hope and trust in God no matter the circumstances. A person who has this attitude is likely to handle stress better, not experience as much physical sickness from stress and be better able to endure hardships.

7. **ESSAY** (5 points): Imagine you have a friend who says he is thinking about suicide. Write an essay explaining how you might deal with the situation. Include in your answer the following:
   - Two signs of suicide that you have noticed in your friend.
   - How his faith in God can make a difference.
   - Where he can turn for help.

Signs of suicide:
  Sudden change in behavior.
  Signs of depression.
  Change of performance in school.
  Loss of interest in friends.
  Giving away of personal items.
  Preoccupation with death, dying or suicide.
  Offhand remarks such as "You may not be seeing me around much."
  Loss of self-esteem.
  Excessive risk-taking.
  Increased drug/alcohol use.

Faith in God can make a difference: Faith changes your perception of the circumstances. God totally understands your feelings and wants you to know He is with you and loves you. Your life does have meaning!

He can turn for help from his parents and family or a teacher, counselor, pastor. Peers are not always a good source of help because they may be going through similar feelings that will reinforce the person's thoughts of suicide.

TOTAL HEALTH

CHAPTER 7: TEST

Unit 2: Mental Health

KEY

100 points

MATCHING (2 points each): For each item on the left column, find the appropriate answer on the right column. Place the letter of the correct answer in the space provided at the left of each item. Each answer may be used only once.

1. _D_ Depression
2. _H_ Stress
3. _E_ Distress
4. _G_ Positive stress
5. _B_ Type A personality
6. _I_ Type B personality
7. _C_ Optimist
8. _F_ Pessimist

A. An intense fear of an object or situation.
B. "Hurried sickness."
C. Someone who looks on the positive side of things.
D. "Sad and blue" feeling.
E. A level of negative stress.
F. Someone who looks on the negative side of things.
G. Challenges a person to meet responsibilities.
H. The body's response to external or internal changes.
I. Someone who is calm and more patient.

FILL IN THE BLANK AND SHORT ANSWER: Answer the following questions (note the points given to each question).

9. No matter what your religious belief, the _Bible_ is a positive prescription for living a healthy life. (2 points)
10. The _"fight or flight"_ response occurs when your body sends out certain hormones to either face your stress or run from it. (2 points)
11. Happiness is a by-product of responding to life from _God's_ perspective. It is not determined by your _circumstances_ but by your _attitudes_ and responses to them. (6 points)
12. "And we know that _God_ causes all things to _work together_ for _good_ to those who _love_ God, to those who are _called_ according to His purpose" Romans 8:28. (10 points)

Chapter Seven, Test Key, page 2 of 3

13. People respond differently to the same stressor. List 4 factors that affect a person's reaction to stress. (4 points)
    1. *The person's age, social status, income, cultural background, stage in life and previous experiences.*
    2. *The circumstances surrounding the situation.*
    3. *How much control the person has or thinks he/she has over the situation.*
    4. *The personality of the person. Type A or B?*
    5. *The person's personal relationship with God.*

14. List 8 effects of negative stress (2 from each category). (8 points)
    PHYSICAL: *loss of appetite, high blood pressure, stroke, headache, anorexia nervosa, loss of menstruation, obesity, cancers of many types, mono, strep, asthma.*
    MENTAL: *Irritability, low self-esteem, depression, lack of creativity, more critical of others and self, grades suffer.*
    SOCIAL: *Uninvolved with friends, angry outbursts, poor time management, lack of communication.*
    SPIRITUAL: *Uninvolved in spiritual activities, no time to pray or read the Word, feelings of guilt and depression, dissatisfaction in life.*

15. List 5 ways to deal with stress. (10 points)
    1. *Eat well.*
    2. *Get plenty of sleep.*
    3. *Laugh it off.*
    4. *Talk things out with someone.*
    5. *Learn to relax.*
    6. *Learn to say "no" to extra activities.*
    7. *Set priorities.*
    8. *Don't let worry drain you.*
    9. *Learn not to procrastinate.*
    10. *Get moving!*
    11. *Time management.*
    12. *Exercise.*
    13. *Write it down: keep a journal.*

16. Explain how too little as well as too much stress can affect a person's performance. (5 points)
    Too little stress can negatively affect performance whether it be an athletic event or academic test. Without stress to motivate you, your performance will be hindered. On the other hand, too much stress can lead to over stimulation and negative stress.

17. Explain why depression is like the "common cold" of mental disorders. (5 points)
    It starts with little sniffles; no one dies of the sniffles. But without proper care, a cold (or depression) can progress from the sniffles to a head cold, to a chest cold and even to pneumonia... plenty of people die of pneumonia. It is also very common and natural to feel depressed at times.

18. Our _attitude_ determines our _action._ (2 points)

19. Explain how your faith in God and His Word can make a difference in the way you handle stress. (5 points)
    - *Trust in God and His Word for the circumstances.*
    - *Knowing He works all things for good.*
    - *Peace in your heart.*

20. **ESSAY** (25 points): Imagine you have a friend who is suffering from depression. He comes to you for help. Write an essay explaining how you might help your friend get out of his depressed state. Include in your essay:
    - Signs of depression that your friend is experiencing.
    - How his faith can make a difference in the way he feels.
    - How his attitude can influence the way he feels.
    - What natural things he can do to help him feel better.

    Possible Answer:
    - *Signs of depression include: inability to sleep, decrease in appetite, feeling bored and unmotivated, losing interest in activities of life, inability to concentrate, feeling of fatigue.*
    - *His faith can make a difference (see answer to #19).*
    - *There is a connection between the attitudes of your mind and your ability to cope with stress. You can experience an overall sense of peace in your life as you develop an attitude of faith and trust (Isaiah 26:3). If you are frustrated and do not trust God with your circumstances you will continue to be depressed and fail to look beyond your circumstances. The principle of positive replacement or having a positive mental attitude can help.*
    - *Natural things you can do to feel better include: Take control of your thoughts, exercise, get moving, use your time wisely, eat well, talk to someone.*

TOTAL HEALTH — CHAPTER 8: QUIZ A

Unit 2: Mental Health

KEY

Sections: 8-1, 8-2
25 points

DEFINE (1 point each): Define the following terms as they are defined in the text.

1. Conduct: *A standard of personal behavior.*
2. Character: *The underlying qualities that are revealed in your actions and attitudes that set you apart. Moral excellence and firmness.*
3. Conviction: *A personal belief upon which certain actions are based. The motivation or reason behind an action.*
4. Biblical conviction: *The framework that holds your Christian walk together.*
5. Conform: *To adapt oneself to prevailing standards or customs: to be or become similar in form or character.*

FILL IN THE BLANK AND SHORT ANSWER: Answer the following questions (note the points given to each question).

6. The _choices_ you are making as a teenager will greatly _affect_ the _lifestyle_ you will have as an _adult._ (4 points)
7. Your _mind_ is never _empty._ The only question is what _fills_ it. (3 points)
8. Explain the G.I.G.O. principle and tell how it ultimately affects your actions. (2 points)
    G.I.G.O. stands for Garbage In, Garbage Out or Good In, Good Out. What goes into your mind will eventually be revealed in your actions. Your mind is like a blank tape that records everything you see, hear, and imagine. It is important to keep your mind on godly things so that your actions will reflect godly character.

9. Explain why it is important to develop personal and biblical convictions. (2 points)
    Personal convictions form the basis for your actions. In turn, your actions eventually become habits. Those habits, either good or bad, influence your lifestyle. It is important to develop strong personal and biblical convictions that will help you lead a lifestyle that is pleasing to God. Also, developing convictions before you are confronted with a situation will help you overcome temptation and doing something you may not want to do.

Copyright © 1995 Susan Boe

10. List 4 of the 7 ways that a person can deal with negative peer pressure. (4 points)
    - *Develop and stand by your convictions.*
    - *Avoid compromising situations.*
    - *Don't give in — not even once.*
    - *Choose your friends wisely.*
    - *Be a positive influence.*
    - *Speak up.*
    - *Run: don't stop and think about it.*

11. **ESSAY** (5 points): You may feel that you are not influenced to conform, but the pressure to be like everyone else can silently affect many areas of your life. Write an essay entitled:

    "How I can overcome the desire to be like everyone else."

    Include in your essay:
    - What is the danger of conforming?
    - What is the strongest pressure to overcome?
    - How can you overcome this pressure?
    - What does God think about conformity? When can conformity be positive?
    - What are three examples where teens may struggle with conformity?

    - *The danger of conforming is that it can keep you from doing what you know is right. Its power is so strong that sometimes you may find yourself caught up in an activity that you never thought you would do.*
    - *The strongest pressure to overcome is peer pressure (or the influence of people on people).*
    - *The power of your mind has much to do with the desire to be like others. The world's influence is very strong, but the Bible can help you overcome that strong negative pressure. Meditate on the Word, think on these things...Philippians 4:8. Be bold and say to others, "I am going to control my behavior, my mind, my body, and my life...When it comes to being moral and obeying God and learning in school and keeping my body clean and healthy, I won't let anyone tell me what to do. If they laugh, let them laugh! I will not conform!"*
    - *The Bible encourages conformity to the image of Christ. Be as much like Christ as possible. Conformity can be positive when the people you desire to be like are living a God-centered life. Most important is to know who Christ is and to desire to be like Him.*
    - *Example teens may struggle with: fashion, speech, attitude to adults, movies, T.V., music, poor behavior in school, drugs, alcohol...*

TOTAL HEALTH

CHAPTER 8: QUIZ B

Unit 2: Mental Health

KEY

Sections: 8-3, 8-4
25 points

FILL IN THE BLANK AND SHORT ANSWER: Answer the following questions (note the points given to each question).

1. "Do not be deceived: _evil (bad)_ company corrupts _good_ habits (I Corinthians 15:33). (2 points)
2. "A new commandment I give to you, that you _love_ one another; as I have _loved_ you, that you also _love_ one another (John 13:34). (3 points)
3. Ask yourself, "what is the _best_ use of my _time_ right now?" (2 points)
4. Explain the following friendship pyramid. Fill in the appropriate level and explain each level of friendship. (4 points)

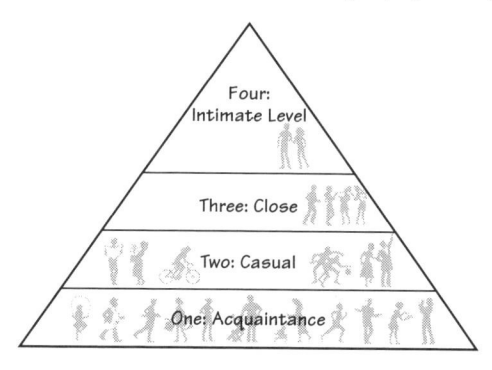

Intimate level: Mutual flow of sharing. This may be a best friend of the same sex, with whom you share all your secrets. As you grow older someone you intend to marry will fill this level.

Close level: few friendships at this level because of the time and emotional connection with them. Share common interests and goals. Example: close friends from class, youth group or sport teams.

Casual level: more friendships but on a casual basis. Not as much in common. Example: students in class whom you spend time with.

Acquaintance level: Many people known by name but do not share common interests. Example: student at school you know but do not spend time with.

Chapter Eight, Quiz B Key, page 2 of 2

5. Explain why it is important to recognize "danger zones" in your friendships. Include in your answer 3 of the 6 questions you should ask yourself when evaluating a friendship. (5 points)

   It is important to recognize "danger zones" in relationships. That is, to be aware when the influence of a friendship is turning negative. You must consider the following when evaluating friendships:
   - *Is this friendship causing me to compromise my values?*
   - *Is this friendship demanding too much of my time?*
   - *Is this friendship causing me to respond negatively to my parents or others in authority?*
   - *Is this friendship focusing on the negatives of others (gossip).*
   - *Is this friendship causing me to like myself more or less?*
   - *Is this friendship pleasing to God?*

6. Earthquakes naturally occur in life. What are the names given to the 3 "earthquakes" discussed in chapter 8? (3 points).
   1. *Emotional Earthquakes.*
   2. *Never Enough Time Earthquakes (or Time Management Earthquakes).*
   3. *The Fear of Failure Earthquakes.*

7. Who usually knows you the best and loves you the most? (1 point)
   Your family

8. **ESSAY** (5 points): Explain why goal setting can positively affect your life. Include in your answer 5 of the 10 principles for goal setting.
   - *Set goals for each area of you life (physical, mental, social and spiritual).*
   - *Keep the goals realistic.*
   - *Keep the goals positive.*
   - *Make a detailed plan for accomplishing each goal…and follow it.*
   - *Make long-range and short-range goals.*
   - *Write your goals down.*
   - *Keep your goals private.*
   - *Do it now!*
   - *Strive for excellence but don't become a perfectionist.*

TOTAL HEALTH — CHAPTER 8: TEST

Unit 2: Mental Health

KEY

100 points

DEFINE (2 points each): Define the following terms as they are defined in the text.

1. Conduct: *A standard of personal behavior.*
2. Character: *The underlying qualities that are revealed in your actions and attitudes that set you apart. Moral excellence and firmness.*
3. Conviction: *A personal belief upon which certain actions are based. The motivation or reason behind an action.*
4. Biblical conviction: *The framework that holds your Christian walk together.*
5. Conform: *To adapt oneself to prevailing standards or customs: to be or become similar in form or character.*

FILL IN THE BLANK AND SHORT ANSWER: Answer the following questions (note the points given to each question).

6. The _choices_ you are making as a teenager will greatly _affect_ the _lifestyle_ you will have as an _adult_. (4 points)
7. Your _mind_ is never _empty._ The only question is what _fills_ it. (3 points)
8. What are the three things by which your lifestyle is measured? (3 points)
    1. *Conduct.*
    2. *Character.*
    3. *Conviction.*

9. Who usually knows you the best and loves you the most? (2 points)
    Your family.

10. "Do not be deceived: _evil (bad)_ company corrupts _good_ habits (I Corinthians 15:33). (2 points)
11. "A new commandment I give to you, that you _love_ one another; as I have _loved_ you, that you also _love_ one another (John 13:34). (3 points)

Copyright © 1995 Susan Boe

12. Fill in the correct words for the following diagram, then explain how it can affect your lifestyle. (5 points)

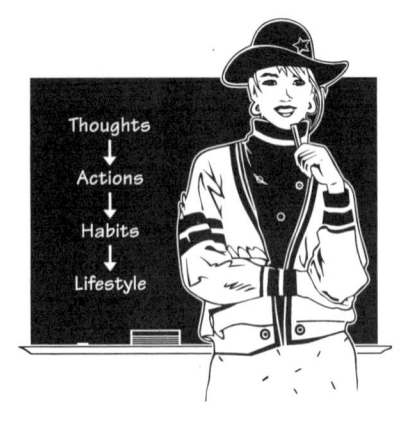

Thoughts → Actions → Habits → Lifestyle

There is a strong connection between your thoughts and your actions. It has been said, "sow a thought, you reap an action: sow an action, you rap a habit: sow a habit, you reap character: sow a character, you reap a destiny." The thought patterns in your life can either result in a negative or positive lifestyle. Self control of your mind and your body requires action. Put off the old self, and put on the new self by renewing the mind (Ephesians 4:22–24). G.I.G.O is a good acronym to remember, Garbage In, Garbage Out or Good In, Good Out. What goes into your mind will eventually be revealed in your actions.

13. A deep but obvious part of who you are is your character. Explain the following diagram as it relates to true character. (10 points)

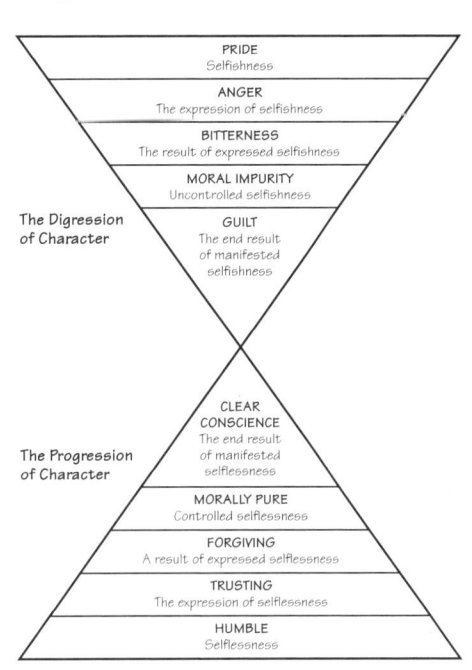

The Digression of Character:
- PRIDE — Selfishness
- ANGER — The expression of selfishness
- BITTERNESS — The result of expressed selfishness
- MORAL IMPURITY — Uncontrolled selfishness
- GUILT — The end result of manifested selfishness

The Progression of Character:
- CLEAR CONSCIENCE — The end result of manifested selflessness
- MORALLY PURE — Controlled selflessness
- FORGIVING — A result of expressed selflessness
- TRUSTING — The expression of selflessness
- HUMBLE — Selflessness

A person does not have to act "religious" to show character. As a matter of fact, it is true selflessness, a humble spirit, that is the foundation of character. There is no acting involved in true character. The chart shows the progression of character and the qualities that develop. A clear conscience is the end result of being selfless, but the end result of being selfish is guilt. Guilt is a very powerful feeling and a heavy burden to carry. Living with a clear conscience allows you to experience true joy. God wants you to develop the character of Christ which is ultimate selflessness.

14. Explain the G.I.G.O. principle and tell how it ultimately affects your actions. (5 points)

G.I.G.O. stands for Garbage In, Garbage Out or Good In, Good Out. What goes into your mind will eventually be revealed in your actions. Your mind is like a blank tape that records everything you see, hear, and imagine. It is important to keep your mind on godly things so that your actions will reflect godly character.

15. Explain why goal setting can positively affect your life. Include in your answer 5 of the 10 principles for goal setting. (5 points)
    - *Set goals for each area of you life (physical, mental, social and spiritual).*
    - *Keep the goals realistic.*
    - *Keep the goals positive.*
    - *Make a detailed plan for accomplishing each goal…and follow it.*
    - *Make long-range and short-range goals.*
    - *Write your goals down.*
    - *Keep your goals private.*
    - *Do it now!*
    - *Strive for excellence but don't become a perfectionist.*

16. Explain why people are afraid to fail, and how people can avoid the "fear of failure" trap. (5 points)

    People are afraid of failure, afraid they will disappoint someone or disappoint God. Fear can paralyze your actions and keep you from reaching your potential. People can avoid this trap by the following:

    1. *Remember that failure or making a mistake is only temporary.*
    2. *God is not in the habit of keeping a record of all your mistakes, so don't you do it.*
    3. *Even if you fail at something, remember, you are not a failure.*
    4. *Failures in life can become positive learning experiences. Learn from your mistakes.*
    5. *Remember, if at first you don't succeed, try, try again!*

17. Life is full of goals, but when life on earth is over only one true goal matters. What is the higher goal everyone should strive to achieve? (3 points)

    To live a life that is pleasing to God.

Chapter Eight, Test Key, page 4 of 5

18. Time management is very important in managing your life. Explain the importance of time management. (10 points) Include in your answer:
    - What is meant by the phrase, "If you fail to plan, then you plan to fail."
    - How to use a fixed commitments chart.
    - Why time management is important to God.
    - Why is self-discipline important in good time management.
    - What role does goal setting have in good time management.

    Possible answer may include:
    - *To manage your time effectively you must have a plan or your time will slip by and you will not accomplish what you had hoped to accomplish. If you set goals it is like setting a course for the direction of your life.*
    - *Place all your fixed commitments in the hours on the chart. For example school hours, job, chores at home, sports or music practice, etc. Then in the space left, you can find slots to accomplish things you thought you did not have time for. You can also find "time wasters" such as those after school hours where you may not be very productive.*
    - *Time management is important to God. It is a resource given to each person. God wants us to use time wisely and productively (Psalm 90:12 Teach us to number our days...Ephesians 5:15,16 See then that you walk circumspectly...).*
    - *Responsible use of your time takes discipline and good planning. Goals can carry you from one success to another. Place God in the control tower of your plans and follow principles of goal setting and you can accomplish much for God!*

19. **ESSAY** (30 points): The desire to conform (to be like others) is very strong. You may feel that you are not influenced by the desire to be like others, but the pressure to conform can silently affect many areas of your life. Write an essay entitled:

"How I can overcome the desire to be like everyone else."

Include in your essay:
- What is the danger of conforming?
- What is the strongest pressure to overcome?
- How can you overcome this pressure?
- The Bible encourages conformity to whose image?
- What are three examples where teens often try to be like others?
- What is your personal feeling about the desire to be like others? When can conformity be positive?

- *The danger of conforming is that it can keep you from doing what you know is right. Its power is so strong that sometimes you may find yourself caught up in an activity that you never thought you would do.*
- *The strongest pressure to overcome is peer pressure (or the influence of people on people).*
- *The power of your mind has much to do with the desire to be like others. The world's influence is very strong, but the Bible can help you overcome that strong negative pressure. Meditate on the Word, think on these things...Philippians 4:8. Be bold and say to others, "I am going to control my behavior, my mind, my body, and my life...When it comes to being moral and obeying God and learning in school and keeping my body clean and healthy, I won't let anyone tell me what to do. If they laugh, let them laugh! I will not conform!"*
- *The Bible encourages conformity to the image of Christ. Be as much like Christ as possible.*
- *Example teens may struggle with: fashion, speech, attitude to adults, movies, T.V., music, poor behavior in school, drugs, alcohol...*
- *Conformity can be positive when the people you desire to be like are living a God-centered life. Most important is to know who Christ is and to desire to be like Him.*

TOTAL HEALTH   CHAPTER 9: QUIZ A

Unit 2: Mental Health

KEY

Sections: 9-1, 9-2, 9-3
25 points

DEFINE (1 point each): Define the following terms as they are defined in the text.

1. Self-image: *The view you have of yourself and the way you believe you are seen by others.*
2. Assume: *To take upon yourself, to take on the particular character that others are saying about you whether it is true or not.*
3. Comfort zone: *An area which a person will not go beyond; a place of security.*
4. Self-talk: *The mental "tape" running in one's mind, repeating all the positive or negative things one hears, sees, reads or imagines.*
5. Countenance: *The face as an indication of mood, emotion, or character.*

FILL IN THE BLANK AND SHORT ANSWER: Answer the following questions (note the points given to each question).

6. When you make *assumptions* about what others think of you, you actually give them *power* to control your *attitude* and *behavior.* (4 points)
7. You cannot control what others will *say* about you, but you can control how you *respond* to it. (2 points)
8. What three attributes are highly valued by society? How can these values give you an unhealthy view of yourself? (4 points)
    1. *Beauty.*
    2. *Physical ability.*
    3. *Intelligence.*

    These qualities are not bad in and of themselves. It is that society places too much importance on these. Man looks on the outer appearance, but God looks at the heart. No one can meet the "perfect" image that society admires. What really matters is what God thinks of you.

9. List 5 of the 8 ways you can improve your self-image. (5 points)
    1. *Get to know the One who made you in His image.*
    2. *Ask for God's help in overcoming your weaknesses.*
    3. *Thank God for the way He has made you.*
    4. *Focus on your strengths.*
    5. *Control your own self-talk.*
    6. *Surround yourself with positive friendships.*
    7. *Change those areas that are changeable.*
    8. *Work at developing inward qualities.*

10. **ESSAY** (5 points): Write an essay responding to the following quote by James Dobson:

    "Most teenagers respect a guy or girl who has the courage to be his own person, even when being teased."

    Accepting the way God has made you is very important. The way you feel about yourself is often portrayed by how you carry yourself. If you lack confidence in who God made you to be then it will show in your countenance. Similarly, if you have a positive view of yourself then your countenance will show this as well.

    Teenagers respect someone who has the courage to stand out of the crowd and be true to the values and beliefs they have about living. If you work more on inward qualities this is naturally attractive to others and also demands a certain respect and admiration from your peers. If you are teased about the way you behave, remember, those inward qualities really do make the best impression in the long run.

TOTAL HEALTH — CHAPTER 9: QUIZ B

Unit 2: Mental Health

KEY

Sections: 9-1, 9-2, 9-3,
25 points

FILL IN THE BLANK AND SHORT ANSWER: Answer the following questions (note the points given to each question).

1. What is the "one-liner" that is a good motto for everyone? (1 point)
   "Put up or Shut up" is a good one-liner. If you don't have anything nice to say, don't say anything at all.

2. What is meant by a self-image "comfort zone"? (2 points)
   A comfort zone is an area which a person will not go beyond. He feels secure to remain in a negative state of mind. It almost becomes a natural condition. A person has a poor self-image and no matter what the circumstances, he remains in that state of mind.

3. Why is remaining in a "comfort zone" dangerous? (2 points)
   It is dangerous to remain in a "comfort zone" because it will keep you from reaching your full potential.

4. What is negative self-talk? (2 points)
   Self-talk is that tape running inside your head repeating all the negative or positive things you hear, see, read or imagine. Negative self-talk is when you hear in your mind the negative input you have received. It becomes so common to you that you believe it.

5. How can a person overcome negative self-talk? Give two examples. (4 points)
   A person can overcome negative self-talk by playing positive words over the negative tapes. The power of the Bible will help to overcome the negative messages in your mind.
   For example: I Samuel 16:7 says: "For man looks on the outward appearance, but the Lord looks at the heart."

6. What three attributes are highly valued by society? How can these values give you an unhealthy view of yourself? (4 points)
   1. *Beauty.*
   2. *Physical ability.*
   3. *Intelligence.*

   These qualities are not bad in and of themselves. It is that society places too much importance on these. Man looks on the outer appearance, but God looks at the heart. No one can meet the "perfect" image that society admires. What really matters is what God thinks of you.

7. You are to be the *reflection* of Him, not in *physical* stature, *talents* or *intelligence*, but in the qualities that *reflect* His nature. (5 points)

8. **ESSAY** (5 points): Write an essay entitled: "The power of the 'one-liner.'"
   Include in your answer:
   - Common ways teenagers tease each other.
   - Give 2 specific examples to show the negative effects of "one-liners."
   - How can teenagers build each other up instead of tearing each other down?
   - What does God think about teasing and the power of words?

   Possible answer may include:
   - *Name calling, appearance, intelligence, athletic inability, popularity.*
   - *One liners leave negative thoughts in a person's memory that are hard to erase. One liners also affect an individual's self-esteem and can negatively affect they way they see themselves for the rest of their lives.*
   - *Teens can offer positive, constructive comments. Teens should try to see one another as God sees. Look past the outer and look at the heart.*
   - *God created each person in His image, as a reflection of Himself. God knows the power of words is very strong and can hurt people. That is why the power of the tongue is discussed in the Bible.*

TOTAL HEALTH

CHAPTER 9: TEST

Unit 2: Mental Health

KEY

100 points

DEFINE (2 points each): Define the following terms as they are defined in the text.

1. Self-image: *The view you have of yourself and the way you believe you are seen by others.*
2. Assume: *To take upon yourself, to take on the particular character that others are saying about you whether it is true or not.*
3. Comfort zone: *An area which a person will not go beyond; a place of security.*
4. Self-talk: *The mental "tape" running in one's mind, repeating all the positive or negative things one hears, sees, reads or imagines.*
5. Countenance: *The face as an indication of mood, emotion, or character.*

FILL IN THE BLANK AND SHORT ANSWER: Answer the following questions (note the points given to each question).

6. When you make _assumptions_ about what others think of you, you actually give them _power_ to control your _attitude_ and _behavior._ (4 points)
7. You cannot control what others will _say_ about you, but you can control how you _respond_ to it. (2 points)
8. What three attributes are highly valued by society? How can these values give you an unhealthy view of yourself? (8 points)
    1. *Beauty.*
    2. *Physical ability.*
    3. *Intelligence.*

    These qualities are not bad in and of themselves. It is that society places too much importance on these. Man looks on the outer appearance, but God looks at the heart. No one can meet the "perfect" image that society admires. What really matters is what God thinks of you.

9. You are to be the _reflection_ of Him, not in _physical_ stature, _talents_ or _intelligence,_ but in the qualities that _reflect_ His nature. (5 points)

10. What is the "one-liner" that is a good motto for everyone? (2 points)

   "Put up or Shut up" is a good one-liner. If you don't have anything nice to say, don't say anything at all.

11. What is negative self-talk? (3 points)

   Self-talk is that tape running inside your head repeating all the negative or positive things you hear, see, read or imagine. Negative self-talk is when you hear in your mind the negative input you have received. It becomes so common to you that you believe it.

12. How can a person overcome negative self-talk? Give two examples. (4 points)

   A person can overcome negative self-talk by playing positive words over the negative tapes. The power of the Bible will help to overcome the negative messages in your mind.
   For example: I Samuel 16:7 says: "For man looks on the outward appearance, but the Lord looks at the heart."

13. List 8 ways you can improve your self-image. (8 points)

   1. Get to know the One who made you in His image.
   2. Ask for God's help in overcoming your weaknesses.
   3. Thank God for the way He has made you.
   4. Focus on your strengths.
   5. Control your own self-talk.
   6. Surround yourself with positive friendships.
   7. Change those areas that are changeable.
   8. Work at developing inward qualities.

14. Explain the meaning of the following verse: "And God created man in His own image, In the image of God He created him; male and female He created them." Genesis 1:27. How should this affect your self-image? (10 points)

   God made you in His image. You are the tangible, visible representation of God. You are to be the reflection of Him. When God sees you, He does not see your weaknesses and faults as you see them. He sees you as a reflection of Himself, Christ in you. The key to understanding this truth is in getting to know the One who created you. Your self-image should improve as you get to know Christ and His character.

15. What is meant by a "comfort zone"? (2 points)
    A comfort zone is an area which a person will not go beyond. He feels secure to remain in a negative state of mind. It almost becomes a natural condition. A person has a poor self-image and no matter what the circumstances, he remains in that state of mind.

16. Why is remaining in a "comfort zone" dangerous? (2 points)
    It is dangerous to remain in a "comfort zone" because it will keep you from reaching your full potential.

17. **ESSAY** (20 points): Write an essay responding to the following quote by James Dobson:

    "Most teenagers respect a guy or girl who has the courage to be his own person, even when being teased."

    Accepting the way God has made you is very important. The way you feel about yourself is often portrayed by how you carry yourself. If you lack confidence in who God made you to be then it will show in your countenance. Similarly, if you have a positive view of yourself then your countenance will show this as well.

    Teenagers respect someone who has the courage to stand out of the crowd and be true to the values and beliefs they have about living. If you work more on inward qualities this is naturally attractive to others and also demands a certain respect and admiration from your peers. If you are teased about the way you behave, remember, those inward qualities really do make the best impression in the long run.

18. **ESSAY** (20 points): Write an essay entitled: "The power of the 'one-liner.'"
    Include in your answer:
    - Common ways teenagers tease each other.
    - Give 2 specific examples to show the negative effects of "one-liners."
    - How can teenagers build each other up instead of tearing each other down?
    - What does God think about teasing and the power of words?

    Answer: Subjective essay: grade on completeness of answer and your measure of the student's understanding of the principle.

TOTAL HEALTH — CHAPTER 10: QUIZ A

Unit 3: Social Health

KEY

Sections: 10-1, 10-2, 10-3
25 points

DEFINE (1 point each): Define the following terms as they are defined in the text.

1. Acne: *A condition that occurs when the pores of the skin become clogged with oil.*
2. Warts: *A growth on the skin caused by a virus.*
3. Dandruff: *Flaking of the outer layer of dead skin cells of the scalp.*
4. Cuticle: *The portion of the fingernail which surrounds the nail and is made up of nonliving skin.*
5. Hangnails: *Splits in the cuticle along the edge of the nail.*

TRUE OR FALSE (1 point each): If the answer is true, put a T to the left of the item number. If the answer is false, put an F to the left of the item number.

- _T_ 6. Good nutrition is a defense against skin problems.
- _F_ 7. A blackhead is created when oil becomes trapped inside a pore.
- _T_ 8. Farsightedness is when a person can see far objects clearly, but close objects appear blurred.
- _T_ 9. The key to good balance is the condition and function of your inner ear.
- _F_ 10. More expensive skin care products mean a better quality product.

FILL IN THE BLANK AND SHORT ANSWER: Answer the following questions (note the points given to each question).

11. The three most important responsibilities you have in caring for your skin are: keep your skin _clean_, keep your skin _moist,_ and keep your skin _protected._ (3 points)
12. Your _personal_ _features_ and _type_ of hair determine whether a cut will look good on your face. (2 points)

Copyright © 1995 Susan Boe

151

13. Why is acne a common problem for teenagers? (3 points)

    The problem of acne may begin during adolescence when the body is going through so many changes. Some hormones cause an increase in the activity of the oil glands. As a result, an oily substance called sebum is made and eventually clogs the pores and causes acne. Although some adults do suffer from breakouts of acne, it usually gets better or disappears altogether after the teen years.

14. You have a friend who wants to stop biting his nails. List 3 of the 8 suggestions to help your friend stop biting his nails. (3 points)
    1. *Make a decision you want to stop.*
    2. *Share that decision with a friend; be accountable.*
    3. *Take pride in the condition of your hands.*
    4. *Keep your nails trimmed and smooth so you will not be tempted to bite them off.*
    5. *Try coating your nails with a bitter tasting nail coating.*
    6. *Try to find out the reason why you bite your nails.*
    7. *Treat yourself to something if you go a month without biting your nails.*
    8. *Limit your biting to one nail.*

15. **ESSAY** (4 points): Write an essay on the natural eyes illustrating a spiritual truth. Give one example of ways your spiritual eyes can be negatively affected. Use the following passage of scripture:

    "The lamp of the body is the eye. If therefore your eye is good, your whole body will be full of light. But if your eye is bad, your whole body will be full of darkness. If therefore the light that is in you is darkness, how great is that darkness!" Matthew 6:22-23.

    Just as it is important to protect your eyes from physical damage, it is important to protect your eyes from negative influences in the world. For example, what you watch on television, what you see in magazines and what you read in books. Protect your spiritual eyes for they are the lamp to the whole body. Negative influences through the eyes cause the whole body to be negatively affected with darkness.

TOTAL HEALTH **CHAPTER 10: QUIZ B**

Unit 3: Social Health

KEY

Sections: 10-4, 10-5
25 points

MATCHING (1 point each): For each item on the left column, find the appropriate answer on the right column. Place the letter of the correct answer in the space provided at the left of each item. Each answer may be used only once.

1. _G_ Premolars
2. _C_ Periodontium
3. _F_ Cavity
4. _J_ Malocclusion
5. _I_ Incisors
6. _H_ Crown
7. _A_ Dentin
8. _K_ Tartar
9. _B_ Canine
10. _E_ Pulp

A. A layer of hard tissue which makes up the root of the tooth.
B. The four pointed teeth responsible for tearing food to prepare it for chewing.
C. The jawbone, gums and ligaments.
D. The part of the tooth that is below the gums.
E. Inside the tooth and consists of blood vessels, nerves and connective tissue.
F. A hole in the tooth.
G. Used to grind and chew the food.
H. The part of the tooth that you can see.
I. The front and center teeth.
J. A condition where the upper and lower teeth do not properly line up.
K. The hard substance that is formed on your teeth.

FILL IN THE BLANK AND SHORT ANSWER: Answer the following questions (note the points given to each question).

11. During a _root canal_ your dentist or specialist will drill a hole in the tooth and remove the exposed root. Then an artificial _crown_ is made to fill the tooth. (2 points)

12. List 3 of the 5 questions you should ask yourself to check your posture. (3 points)
    1. *Do you lean on an elbow on your desk while in class?*
    2. *Do you find yourself tipping your chair either forward or backward to change positions?*
    3. *Do you find yourself tired and falling asleep in class?*
    4. *Do you carry your books in a bookbag on one shoulder on the same side of your body?*
    5. *Do you lean over without bending your knees and keeping your back straight when you pick up something?*

13. What are 3 things to remember when you are buying a pair of shoes? (3 points)
    1. *Choose shoes that are flexible and supple but firm in the arch. Pick up a shoe and bend it. Does it feel flexible?*
    2. *Choose shoes that have laces or adjustable straps because they can keep the foot from sliding.*
    3. *Choose shoes that are at least half an inch longer than the feet and wide enough to allow the toes to move comfortably.*
    4. *Choose shoes only after you walk around in them. Remember to put on both shoes at the same time. One foot may fit differently in the shoes.*

14. Your posture is a reflection of your __mood__ and your __self-image.__ (2 points)

15. **ESSAY** (5 points): Taking good care of your teeth now at a young age is very important. Write an essay explaining why it is important to take good care of your teeth and gums. Include in your answer:
    - What are the problems that may occur if you do not take good care of your teeth and gums?
    - What are the "do's" of tooth care?
    - What are the "don'ts" of tooth care?

    - *If you do not take good care of your teeth and gums from an early age, you will develop problems as an adult. Gingivitis (gum disease), periodontal disease (more severe gum disease), cavities, root canals, crowns, plaque can form and tartar will build up.*

Do's:
- *Do brush regularly after every meal if possible, at least twice a day.*
- *Do avoid sugary foods.*
- *Do replace your toothbrush after you have had a cold or flu.*
- *Do floss your teeth after you brush rather than before.*
- *Do have regular dental check-ups, every six months or once a year.*
- *Do use a toothpaste that has fluoride.*

Don'ts:
- *Don't overbrush your teeth.*
- *Don't use toothpastes that claim to whiten your teeth.*
- *Don't smoke or use chewing tobacco.*

TOTAL HEALTH — CHAPTER 10: TEST

Unit 3: Social Health

KEY

100 points

DEFINE (2 points each): Define the following terms as they are defined in the text.

1. Acne: *A condition that occurs when the pores of the skin become clogged with oil.*
2. Warts: *A growth on the skin caused by a virus.*
3. Dandruff: *Flaking of the outer layer of dead skin cells of the scalp.*
4. Cuticle: *The portion of the fingernail which surrounds the nail and is made up of nonliving skin.*
5. Hangnails: *Splits in the cuticle along the edge of the nail.*
6. Keratin: *A tough, dead material that your nails are made of.*
7. Nearsightedness: *A person can see close objects clearly, but distant objects appear blurred.*
8. Farsightedness: *A person can see far objects clearly, but close objects appear blurred.*
9. Gingivitis: *A gum disease caused by a build up of plaque and tarter on the teeth.*
10. Plaque: *A grainy, sticky coating that is constantly forming on your teeth.*

TRUE OR FALSE (2 points each): If the answer is true, put a T to the left of the item number. If the answer is false, put an F to the left of the item number.

_T_ 11. Good nutrition is a defense against skin problems.
_T_ 12. A whitehead is created when oil becomes trapped inside a pore.
_F_ 13. Although comfort is important in shoes, style should have high priority.
_T_ 14. The key to good balance is the condition and function of your inner ear.
_F_ 15. You can never overbrush your teeth.

FILL IN THE BLANK: Fill in the space with the appropriate answer to complete the statement (note the points given to each question).

16. During a _root canal_ your dentist or specialist will drill a hole in the tooth and remove the exposed root. Then an artificial _crown_ is made to fill the tooth. (2 points)

17. An _orthodontist_ is a dentist who specializes in treating irregularities in the teeth. (1 point)
18. _Balance_ or equilibrium is your ability to remain steady and in control of your body. (1 point)
19. _Motion sickness_ is the feeling of dizziness and/or nausea while riding in a car, boat, or airplane. (1 point)
20. Your posture is a reflection of your _mood_ and your _self-image_. (2 points)
21. The three most important responsibilities you have in caring for your skin are: keep your skin _clean,_ keep your skin _moist,_ and keep your skin _protected._ (3 points)
22. Your _personal features_ and _type_ of hair determine whether a cut will look good on your face. (2 points)

MATCHING (1 point each): For each item on the left column, find the appropriate answer on the right column. Place the letter of the correct answer in the space provided at the left of each item. Each answer may be used only once.

23. _C_ Crown
24. _F_ Cavity
25. _E_ Tartar
26. _B_ Pulp

27. _A_ Root
28. _H_ Dentin
29. _D_ Malocclusion
30. _I_ Periodontium

A. The part of the tooth that is below the gum.
B. Consists of blood vessels, nerves and tissue.
C. The part of the tooth that you can see.
D. A condition where the upper and lower teeth do not line up properly.
E. The hard substance that is formed on your teeth.
F. A hole in the tooth.
G. The front and center teeth.
H. A layer of hard tissue which makes up the root of the tooth.
I. The jawbone, gums and ligaments.

SHORT ANSWER: Answer the following questions (note the points given to each question).

31. Why is acne a common problem for teenagers? (5 points)
    The problem of acne may begin during adolescence when the body is going through so many changes. Some hormones cause an increase in the activity of the oil glands. As a result, an oily substance called sebum is made and eventually clogs the pores and causes acne. Although some adults do suffer from breakouts of acne, it usually gets better or disappears altogether after the teen years.

32. You have a friend who wants to stop biting his nails. List 5 of the 8 suggestions to help your friend stop biting his nails. (5 points)
    1. *Make a decision you want to stop.*
    2. *Share that decision with a friend; be accountable.*
    3. *Take pride in the condition of your hands.*
    4. *Keep your nails trimmed and smooth so you will not be tempted to bite them off.*
    5. *Try coating your nails with a bitter tasting nail coating.*
    6. *Try to find out the reason why you bite your nails.*
    7. *Treat yourself to something if you go a month without biting your nails.*
    8. *Limit your biting to one nail.*

33. Using headphones to listen to music can be enjoyable, but the risks are great if you do not use caution. What are 2 risks of using headphones? (4 points)
    1. *Can keep you inattentive to the sounds around you. Traffic, phone calls.*
    2. *Can damage your hearing if they are used for extended periods of time and if the sound is too loud.*

34. List 4 of the 5 questions you should ask yourself to check your posture. (4 points)
    1. *Do you lean on an elbow on your desk while in class?*
    2. *Do you find yourself tipping your chair either forward or backward to change positions?*
    3. *Do you find yourself tired and falling asleep in class?*
    4. *Do you carry your books in a bookbag on one shoulder on the same side of your body?*
    5. *Do you lean over without bending your knees and keeping your back straight when you pick up something?*

35. What are 3 things to remember when you are buying a pair of shoes? (3 points)
    1. *Choose shoes that are flexible and supple but firm in the arch. Pick up a shoe and bend it. Does it feel flexible?*
    2. *Choose shoes that have laces or adjustable straps because they can keep the foot from sliding.*
    3. *Choose shoes that are at least half an inch longer than the feet and wide enough to allow the toes to move comfortably.*
    4. *Choose shoes only after you walk around in them. Remember to put on both shoes at the same time. One foot may fit differently in the shoes.*

36. What are the 4 suggestions for taking good care of your skin from the "inside-out"? Good nutrition as a defense against skin problems.
    1. *Vitamin C: helps produce collagen and gives skin its elasticity.*
    2. *Vitamin E: helps to fight against the effects of pollution and ultraviolet rays.*
    3. *Beta-carotene: good in the fight against acne.*
    4. *Drink plenty of water: helps your skin get enough moisture and cleanses your body.*

37. **ESSAY**(15 points): Taking good care of your teeth now at a young age is very important. Write an essay explaining why it is important to take good care of your teeth and gums. Include in your answer:
    - What are the problems that may occur if you do not take good care of your teeth and gums? (5 points)
    - What are the "do's" of tooth care? (5 points)
    - What are the "don'ts" of tooth care? (5 points)

    - *If you do not take good care of your teeth and gums from an early age, you will develop problems as an adult. Gingivitis (gum disease), periodontal disease (more severe gum disease), cavities, root canals, crowns, plaque can form and tartar will build up.*

Do's:
- *Do brush regularly after every meal if possible, at least twice a day.*
- *Do avoid sugary foods.*
- *Do replace your toothbrush after you have had a cold or flu.*
- *Do floss your teeth after you brush rather than before.*
- *Do have regular dental check-ups, every six months or once a year.*
- *Do use a toothpaste that has flouride.*

Don'ts:
- *Don't overbrush your teeth.*
- *Don't use toothpastes that claim to whiten your teeth.*
- *Don't smoke or use chewing tobacco.*

38. **ESSAY** (15 points): The Bible uses the natural eye to illustrate a spiritual truth. Include in your answer:
- What is meant by your "spiritual eyes"? (5 points)
- Give 2 examples of ways your spiritual eyes can be negatively affected. (2 points)
- Explain the meaning of the scripture in Matthew 6:22-23. (8 points)

"The lamp of the body is the eye. If therefore your eye is good, your whole body will be full of light. But if your eye is bad, your whole body will be full of darkness. If therefore the light that is in you is darkness, how great is that darkness!" Matthew 6:22-23

> *Just as it is important to protect your eyes from physical damage, it is important to protect your eyes from negative influences in the world. For example, what you watch on television, what you see in magazines and what you read in books. Protect your spiritual eyes for they are the lamp to the whole body. Negative influences through the eyes cause the whole body to be negatively affected with darkness.*

TOTAL HEALTH **CHAPTER 11: QUIZ A**

Unit 3: Social Health

KEY

Sections: 11-1, 11-2
25 points

SHORT ANSWER: Answer the following questions (note the points given to each question).

1. List 3 reasons why teenagers are more likely to take unnecessary risks. (3 points)
    1. *Teens believe that they are in the peak of health; they are indestructible.*
    2. *Teens do not think about the possible consequences; as a result they do not make careful decisions.*
    3. *Teens are "thrill-seekers."*
    4. *Teens do not want to appear cowardly to their friends.*
    5. *Teens are unwilling to face the fact that there is a possibility of danger.*

2. Before you decide to participate in a "questionable" activity, list 3 questions you should ask yourself. (3 points)
    1. *How much is known about the activity (what exactly are you going to do).*
    2. *What risks are involved?*
    3. *What can I do to reduce those risks or substitute a less risky activity?*
    4. *If I cannot reduce the risks or substitute a less risky activity, is the activity still worth doing?*

3. What is meant by the phrase, "the Lord's protection is not absolute." (2 points)
    You must take responsibility for your actions and decisions. When you lack wisdom you are more likely to participate in questionable activities. Would God be pleased to come along with you while you participate in this activity?

4. Sometimes your own personal safety is threatened by crime. List 3 precautions you can take to help you avoid being a victim of criminal action. (3 points)
    1. *Travel in groups.*
    2. *Keep your doors and windows locked (car included).*
    3. *Avoid dark streets and unpopulated areas.*
    4. *Always look and ask who is at your door before opening it.*
    5. *Avoid interactions with strangers.*
    6. *Avoid giving any information over the phone to a stranger.*
    7. *If something "feels" wrong, find an adult or police officer.*

5. What is "date rape" and what precautions should a person take to avoid this from happening? (4 points)

   Date rape occurs when the victim is forced to have sexual intercourse by someone on a date. The best precaution is to avoid getting into a situation where you find yourself alone, in a private area where your date could take advantage of you. Never feel you must give in to this person because you are "friends."

6. What is the first aid for a person who you suspect has swallowed a poison? (4 points)
   1. *Call the Poison Control Center. Take the container with you to the phone so you will have the information for the operator.*
   2. *Call 911 and tell them that you have called the poison control center.*
   3. *Save the container of substance and give it to the medical team when they arrive.*
   4. *Wipe the victims mouth clean.*

7. List 3 fire safety precautions for the home. (3 points)
   1. *Be careful while cooking. Never leave the area while you are cooking. Turn pot handles inward to avoid knocking them over. If a grease fire occurs, carefully cover the pan with a lid then turn off the burner. Do not use water to put out a grease fire.*
   2. *Keep electrical wiring in good working order. Do not overload extension cords.*
   3. *Keep matches and lighters out of the hands of children.*
   4. *Throw out old newspapers and other combustibles.*
   5. *Keep space heaters at least three feet from anything that can burn. Always turn them off when you leave your home.*

8. Bicycle riding has become a very popular mode of transportation. List 3 safety rules of the road for bicycle riders. (3 points)
   1. *Always ride on the right side of the street (with the flow of traffic).*
   2. *Always obey the traffic signals.*
   3. *Always look back over your shoulder frequently and pay extra attention when passing driveways.*
   4. *Always use proper hand signals for turning. Yield to cars and pedestrians.*
   5. *Always keep your bike in good working condition.*
   6. *Always wear a helmet.*
   7. *Always use reflectors and reflective clothes when riding.*

TOTAL HEALTH

CHAPTER 11: QUIZ B

Unit 3: Social Health

KEY

Sections: 11-3, 11-4
25 points

SHORT ANSWER: Answer the following questions (note the points given to each question).

1. What is the definition of first aid? (1 point)
   The immediate care given to a person who has been injured or has been suddenly taken ill until qualified medical care can be supplied.

2. The person giving first aid is called the _first_ - _aider._ (1 point)
3. First aid begins with _action_. (1 point)
4. When you come upon the seen of an accident, the first thing you must do is survey the situation. What does it mean to survey the situation? (2 points)
   To survey the situation means to quickly view all of the victims and their conditions as you see it.

5. Once you have surveyed the situation, you should do the following in the order they are listed. (4 points)
   #1. Rescue the victim.
   #2. Check the victim's breathing.
   #3. Control severe bleeding.
   #4. Get help!

6. Number the following steps in order of proper action (1 = what to do first). (4 points)
   _3_ Elevate the wound.
   _1_ Take immediate action.
   _4_ Use a pressure point.
   _2_ Apply direct pressure.

7. What are the 3 classifications of burns. Describe the treatment for each. (6 points)

Classification	Treatment
A. First degree burn	A. Hold the burn under cold water, elevate the area above the heart
B. Second degree burn	B. Do the same as for first degree but also remember not to break the blisters. See a doctor if the burn covers more than two inches or becomes infected.
C. Third degree burn	C. Get medical care immediately. You may cover the area with a sterile dressing. Treat the person for shock.

8. What are the ABC's of artificial respiration? Describe each. (6 points)

Airway
 a. Open the airway by tilting the head backward. Clear out the mouth of any object.
 b. Look, listen and feel: Look for chest to rise, listen for exhalation, feel for breath.

Breathing
 a. Pinch nostrils with hand resting on forehead.
 b. Take a deep breath and with your mouth open widely, seal your mouth tightly over the victim's mouth. Give four quick breaths.
 c. Look, listen and feel.
 d. Repeat if not breathing, giving about 12 breaths per minute.
 e. Repeat steps if breathing does not start.

Circulation
 a. Check for pulse on side of neck.
 b. If no pulse is felt administer CPR.
 c. Re-check pulse and breathing every minute.

TOTAL HEALTH

CHAPTER 11: TEST

Unit 3: Social Health

KEY

100 points

FILL IN THE BLANK AND SHORT ANSWER: Answer the following questions (note the points given to each question).

1. List 3 reasons why teenagers are more likely to take unnecessary risks. (3 points)
    1. *Teens believe that they are in the peak of health; they are indestructible.*
    2. *Teens do not think about the possible consequences; as a result they do not make careful decisions.*
    3. *Teens are "thrill-seekers."*
    4. *Teens do not want to appear cowardly to their friends.*
    5. *Teens are unwilling to face the fact that there is a possibility of danger.*

2. Before you decide to participate in a "questionable" activity, list 3 questions you should ask yourself. (3 points)
    1. *How much is known about the activity (what exactly are you going to do).*
    2. *What risks are involved?*
    3. *What can I do to reduce those risks or substitute a less risky activity?*
    4. *If I cannot reduce the risks or substitute a less risky activity, is the activity still worth doing?*

3. The Lord's _protection_ is not _absolute._ (2 points)
4. What is "date rape" and what precautions should a person take to avoid this from happening? (5 points)
    Date rape occurs when the victim is forced to have sexual intercourse by someone on a date. The best precaution is to avoid getting into a situation where you find yourself alone, in a private area where your date could take advantage of you. Never feel you must give in to this person because you are "friends."

5. Accidents _will_ but do not _have to_ happen. (2 points)
6. Everyone should know this rule if your clothes catch on fire, _stop,_ _drop_ and _roll._ (2 points)

7. What is the definition of first aid? (2 points)
    The immediate care given to a person who has been injured or has been suddenly taken ill until qualified medical care can be supplied.

8. The person giving first aid is called the __first__ - __aider.__ (2 points)
9. First aid begins with __action__. (2 points)
10. What are the 3 classifications of burns. Describe the treatment for each. (6 points)

    <u>Classification</u>   <u>Treatment</u>
    A. *First degree burn*   A. *Hold the burn under cold water, elevate the area above the heart*

    B. *Second degree burn*   B. *Do the same as for first degree but also remember not to break the blisters. See a doctor if the burn covers more than two inches or becomes infected.*

    C. *Third degree burn*   C. *Get medical care immediately. You may cover the area with a sterile dressing. Treat the person for shock.*

11. What are the ABC's of artificial respiration? Describe each. (6 points)

    Airway
    a. *Open the airway by tilting the head backward. Clear out the mouth of any object.*
    b. *Look, listen and feel: Look for chest to rise, listen for exhalation, feel for breath.*

    Breathing
    a. *Pinch nostrils with hand resting on forehead.*
    b. *Take a deep breath and with your mouth open widely, seal your mouth tightly over the victim's mouth. Give four quick breaths.*
    c. *Look, listen and feel.*
    d. *Repeat if not breathing, giving about 12 breaths per minute.*
    e. *Repeat steps if breathing does not start.*

    Circulation
    a. *Check for pulse on side of neck.*
    b. *If no pulse is felt administer CPR.*
    c. *Re-check pulse and breathing every minute.*

12. You are babysitting a 3 year old. While you are watching television you do not notice that the child walks out of the room. When the child enters the room you notice white powder around her lips and mouth. She is saying it hurts. You walk into the kitchen and notice the dishwashing detergent is spilled on the floor.

    What can you assume from the situation? What are you going to do to administer first aid to this child? You may add any details to explain your situation. (5 points)

    - *The child has placed the dishwashing detergent in her mouth.*
    - *Call the Poison Control Center immediately. Do exactly what they say. Take the substance to the phone with you so you have the information to give to the operator.*
    - *Call the 911 emergency operator and tell them you have called the Poison Control Center.*
    - *Save the detergent box and give it to the medical team when they arrive.*
    - *Wipe the mouth clean: take a clean, moist cloth and wipe the mouth of the victim clean of excess substance around or inside the mouth.*
    - *Keep the child calm and quiet. Call the parents.*

13. You are playing tennis with a friend. It is extremely hot and you have been playing for a long time. When you have taken water breaks your friend has not. Suddenly she collapses on the tennis court. She is pale and her skin is clammy. She is sweating profusely. No one else is around. You must first determine what she is suffering from, is this heatstroke or heat exhaustion?

    What is your friend suffering from? Explain the proper first aid steps for that condition. You may add any details to explain your situation. (5 points)

    - *Heat exhaustion.*
    - *Move her to the shade or cooler area.*
    - *Lay her down if she is not already.*
    - *Loosen her clothing.*
    - *Elevate her feet.*
    - *Give her sips of cool water.*
    - *You can also fan her or use cool, wet cloths to cool her body temperature.*

TOTAL HEALTH — CHAPTER 12: QUIZ A

Unit 3: Social Health

KEY

Sections: 12-1, 12-2, 12-3,
25 points

FILL IN THE BLANK AND SHORT ANSWER: Answer the following questions (note the points given to each question).

1. Define the word attitude. (1 point)
    An attitude is a feeling or emotion toward something.

2. How does society's message about success differ from God's message? (4 points)
    Your lifestyle may seem directly opposite to what society portrays as "successful." Pride, position, and power is the message that society wants you to hear and follow. These words speak selfish ambition and defeat. God has a different message — love, submission and obedience. These words speak Godly ambition and victory in life.

3. God has a special __plan__. No one can __stop__ it, but many can __miss__ it! (3 points)

4. List 5 of the responsibilities a Christian has in living as a soldier of Christ. (5 points)
    - *Love God.*
    - *Love one another.*
    - *Extend the Kingdom.*
    - *Obey His commandments.*
    - *Be an example in word and deed.*

5. Explain what it means to be a good steward of your physical body. Why is this important? (2 points).
    Good nutrition, physical exercise and a thankful heart help the physical body be strong. The better physical health that you experience, the more energy you will have to give to God and to others.

6. John Donne said, "No man is an island." What does this mean? What is your social responsibility? (2 points)
    No person can live without touching the lives of others. No matter how hard you try, you cannot live a solitary life. God has called every believer to show the love of God. This is the foundation of your social responsibility.

Copyright © 1995 Susan Boe

7. Explain what it means to shirk, shelve, shoulder and shed your responsibilities. And what is the result of having these attitudes? (8 points)
    - *TO SHIRK:* *To avoid performing an obligation or duty. Results in lack of maturity.*
    - *TO SHELVE:* *To put responsibilities off the "to do" list and on to the "waiting" list. Results in missing out on what God wants to do in your life now.*
    - *TO SHOULDER:* *To assume the burden alone. The result is getting wounded and then burn out from exhaustion.*
    - *TO SHED:* *To rid yourself of the responsibilities. The result is never reaching your destiny because you give back to God the things He wants you to accomplish.*

TOTAL HEALTH

CHAPTER 12: QUIZ B

Unit 3: Social Health

KEY

Section: 12-4
25 points

MATCHING (1 point each): For each item on the left column, find the appropriate answer on the right column. Place the letter of the correct answer in the space provided at the left of each item. Each answer may be used only once.

1. __B__ Pollution
2. __D__ Acid rain
3. __F__ Biodegradable

4. __G__ Ozone layer
5. __A__ Greenhouse effect
6. __C__ Environmentalist

A. Warming of the earth's temperature.
B. Contamination
C. Someone who is concerned about the quality of the environment.
D. Contains pollutants from the air.
E. 70% of the earth's surface is covered with this.
F. Able to be broken down in water without causing a problem.
G. A form of oxygen that is formed naturally in the upper atmosphere.

SHORT ANSWER: Answer the following questions (note the points given to each question).

7. Being wise with your waste is very important. What 3 terms are used to describe this. Give an example for each. (6 points)
   1. *Reduce: to decrease in size, amount, extent or number. For example, purchase things that are packaged with a refill system: laundry detergent.*
   2. *Reuse: to use something over for another purpose. Reuse your paper sack from the grocery store.*
   3. *Recycle: a process that takes material that would otherwise be garbage and regain it for human use. Example: plastics, newspaper.*

8. List 5 of the 10 consumer skills that can make you a better steward of your money. (5 points)
    - *Use your money wisely, getting the most out of your dollar.*
    - *Buy goods and services that help you have good health.*
    - *Do your homework! Comparison shop.*
    - *If you have a problem with goods or services, don't ignore it, get help.*
    - *Take good care of what you have already.*
    - *Be a good influence on your family and peers.*
    - *Avoid peer pressure to conform to what others are buying.*
    - *Avoid buying when you are in a hurry.*
    - *Avoid grocery shopping when you are hungry or without a list.*
    - *Pray for wisdom when spending your money.*

9. Give 3 examples of how advertisers try to get teens to buy certain products. (3 points)
    - *Coke: Testimonials from famous people.*
    - *Lifestyle appeal: a commercial for a car or product that looks like you will have fun if you buy it.*
    - *False image appeal: If you use this shampoo, your hair will look like this.*

10. **ESSAY** (5 points): A citizen is a person living in a town or country who owes allegiance to a government and is entitled to the rights, privileges and protection of it. You are a citizen of the earthly government that rules your country, but you are also a citizen of the Kingdom of God. God wants you to be a responsible citizen. Write an essay entitled:

    "How I can be a responsible citizen to God and to my country."

    - *Becoming a knowledgable voter when I am of age.*
    - *Writing letters to the appropriate governing officials of issues you are concerned about.*
    - *Praying for your country.*
    - *Obeying God's laws.*
    - *Influence society for God.*

TOTAL HEALTH   CHAPTER 12: TEST

Unit 3: Social Health

KEY

100 points

DEFINE (2 points each): Define the following terms as they are defined in the text.

1. Attitude: *A feeling or emotion toward something.*
2. Steward: *A manager, supervisor, superintendent; to hold the office of oversight of another's property or affairs.*
3. Environmentalist: *Someone who is concerned about the quality of the environment.*
4. Acid rain: *The rain that contains pollutants.*
5. Ozone layer: *A form of oxygen that is formed naturally in the upper atmosphere.*

TRUE OR FALSE (2 points each): If the answer is true, put a T to the left of the item number. If the answer is false, put an F to the left of the item number.

- _F_ 6. The majority of pollution on the earth is made up of natural gases.
- _F_ 7. The greenhouse effect is a cooling of the earth's temperature.
- _T_ 8. As a result of the decrease in the ozone layer, the sun's rays are more dangerous.
- _T_ 9. Biodegradable products can be broken down by water without a problem.
- _F_ 10. Water shortages are not a problem because more than 70% of the earth is covered with water.

FILL IN THE BLANK AND SHORT ANSWER: Answer the following questions (note the points given to each question).

11. God has a special _plan_. No one can _stop_ it, but many can _miss_ it! (3 points)
12. "No man is an _island,_ entire of itself; every man is a piece of the Continent, a part of the _main_." John Donne (2 points)
13. Freedom is not really _valued_ for its true worth unless it is _earned._ (2 points)
14. Although your degree(s) in school will not be among your _"heavenly treasures,"_ it is a means to fulfilling your _destiny_ in God and _influencing_ society for Christ. (3 points)

15. List 5 of the responsibilities a Christian has in living as a soldier of Christ. (5 points)
    - *Love God.*
    - *Love one another.*
    - *Extend the Kingdom.*
    - *Obey His commandments.*
    - *Be an example in word and deed.*

16. Explain what it means to be a good steward of your physical body. Why is this important? (2 points)

    Good nutrition, physical exercise and a thankful heart help the physical body be strong. The better physical health that you experience the more energy you will have to give to God and to others.

17. What is your social responsibility according to God? (2 points)

    God has called every believer to show the love of God.

18. Name and define the 3 terms used to describe what you can do to be wise with your waste. Give one example for each. (6 points)
    1. *Reduce: to decrease in size, amount, extent or number. For example, purchase things that are packaged with a refill system: laundry detergent.*
    2. *Reuse: to use something over for another purpose. Reuse your paper sack from the grocery store.*
    3. *Recycle: a process that takes material that would otherwise be garbage and regain it for human use. Example: plastics, newspaper.*

19. Give 4 examples of how advertisers try to get people to buy their products. (4 points)
    - *Bandwagon: "everybody's doing it." Join the Pepsi Generation.*
    - *Snob Appeal: "eat imperial and feel like a king."*
    - *Glittering generality appeal: "end all headaches."*
    - *Testimonial appeal: Michael Jordan and basketball shoes.*
    - *False image appeal: "if you use this shampoo, your hair will look like this."*
    - *Humor: "I can't believe I ate the whole thing."*
    - *Sex appeal: smoking, car and exercise video commercials.*
    - *Lifestyle appeal: people having a good time when they use their product.*
    - *Scientific evidence appeal: "in a recent hospital survey…"*

20. What is exploitation of consumers? Give 2 examples of exploitation. (3 points)
    Exploitation means to make unethical use for one's own advantage or profit. For example Saturday morning cartoons directed toward children, or disc jockeys trying to get you to listen to them. Stores that draw you in on "sales" and then raise their prices on other items.

21. List 3 things to remember when choosing a health-care provider. (3 points)
    - *Read thoroughly and understand your health insurance information.*
    - *Ask a friend or family member.*
    - *Check the name of several doctors with your insurance.*
    - *Call the service and ask questions over the phone.*
    - *Call for a consultation.*
    - *Prepare a list of questions for the doctor.*

22. **ESSAY**: (25 points): Write an essay entitled:
    "How I can be a good steward of my money."

Include in your essay an explanation of the following verse: (5 points)

"He who is faithful in a very little thing is faithful also in much: and he who is unrighteous in a very little thing is unrighteous also in much. If therefore you have not been faithful in the use of unrighteous mammon, who will entrust the true riches to you? And if you have not been faithful in the use of that which is another's, who will give you that which is your own?" Luke 16: 10-12

- How this verse can relate to a teenager. (5 points)
- 5 influences that affect your buying a certain product. (5 points)
- A minimum of 5 of the 10 consumer skills that can make you a better steward of your money. (5 points)
- Personal examples where you can be a better steward of your money. (5 points)

A person who can take responsibility of the little things now will be given greater responsibility. With money, if you are not a faithful steward of what little you have now or of another's money (i.e., your parents), how can you be trusted more? Teens begin to take responsibility in the areas of money, for example, as they get a job or receive money from their parents to purchase things. They need to be good stewards of what they have.

Influences that affect buying choices:
- *The cost.*
- *The advertising.*
- *The knowledge and skill of sales person.*
- *The features of the product.*
- *The quality.*
- *The convenience.*
- *The warranty or guarantee.*
- *The peer pressure.*

Consumer skills:
- *Use your money wisely, getting the most out of your dollar.*
- *Buy goods and services that help you have good health.*
- *Do your homework! comparison shop.*
- *If you have a problem with goods or services, don't ignore it, get help.*
- *Take good care of what you have already.*
- *Be a good influence on your family and peers*
- *Avoid peer pressure to conform to what others are buying.*
- *Avoid buying when you are in a hurry.*
- *Avoid grocery shopping when you are hungry or without a list.*
- *Pray for wisdom when spending your money.*

23. **ESSAY**: (20 points): There are 5 possible attitudes one can have toward responsibility. Write an essay explaining each attitude.
   Include in your essay:
   - The definition of responsibility according to Archibald Naismith and how this definition can apply to your life. (5 points)
   - The meaning of each attitude. (5 points)
   - The result of having each attitude. (5 points)
   - What is the best attitude to have and why. (5 points)

   - *Responsibility is: Your response to God's ability.*
TO SHIRK:	*To avoid performing an obligation or duty. Results in lack of maturity.*
TO SHELVE:	*To put responsibilities off the "to do" list and on to the "waiting" list. Results in missing out on what God wants to do in your life now.*
TO SHOULDER:	*To assume the burden alone. The result is getting wounded and then burn out from exhaustion.*
TO SHED:	*To rid yourself of the responsibilities. The result is never reaching your destiny because you give back to God the things He wants you to accomplish.*
TO SHARE:	*To partake of, use, experience or enjoy with others. You are better able to reach your potential because you gain strength and guidance from others.*

   - *The best attitude to have is to SHARE responsibility because the army of God is strengthened by every one taking on only the responsibilities they are to have (not more).*
     People gain protection and wisdom working with others and sharing the load.

TOTAL HEALTH

CHAPTER 13: QUIZ A

Unit 3: Social Health

KEY

Section: 13-1
25 points

FILL IN THE BLANK AND SHORT ANSWER: Answer the following questions (note the points given to each question).

1. Explain how your mind is like a library. (3 points)
    Your brain is like a library; it has the ability to store information. Volumes of information are stored on the "shelves" of your mind. Whatever you receive in your mind, you first categorize, and then store these volumes. When you need the information, you draw from it to make decisions. Not everyone's library looks the same or holds the same information.

2. How has the Creator made the human race unique from the creation of other living beings? (3 points)
    God has given humans volumes of common sense and wisdom. People have the ability to know where they came from, know where they want to go, how they want to live and what they want to do. People also have the capacity to know right from wrong.

3. Explain why people often have a "right now" mentality. How can this mentality be dangerous? (3 points)
    Society is a "right now" society. You don't always know the long-term results of your decisions. Furthermore, the benefits of making right choices are not always instantaneous. This can be a dangerous attitude because you may do things that will negatively affect your life because you do not see the consequences right away. Right choices often require waiting for long-term results.

4. One aspect of your __maturity__ is the ability to make __wise decisions.__ (2 points)
5. Remember, maturity is not something you "arrive at" during your lifetime, __maturity__ is a __process.__ (2 points)
6. What is puberty? (2 points)
    The stage of growth and development at which males and females become physically able to reproduce.

7. List 5 signs of maturity (<u>not</u> including physical signs of maturity). (5 points)
   - *Has self-control.*
   - *Recognizes godly values: makes good judgments.*
   - *Recognizes the importance of setting goals.*
   - *Stands up for what is right even when persecuted.*
   - *Assumes responsibility for actions.*
   - *Avoids compromising situations.*
   - *Avoids being judgmental or critical of others.*
   - *Is able to be trusted.*
   - *Respects others: forms mature relationships.*
   - *Has more concern for others: not so self-centered.*

8. Why does God place boundaries in your life? (3 points)
   God places boundaries in your life not to see you fail or to have you be unhappy, but to protect you.

9. God's laws are <u>*realistic*</u> for your life. (1 point)

10. Spiritual maturity is the area of maturity that will take you into <u>*eternity.*</u> (1 point)

TOTAL HEALTH — CHAPTER 13: QUIZ B

Unit 3: Social Health

KEY

Section: 13-2
25 points

SHORT ANSWER: Answer the following questions (note the points given to each question).

1. Explain the meaning of the phrase, "abstinence is not the only goal." (2 points)
    Many young people go "too far" without "going all the way." That is, they engage in sexual activity but do not have intercourse. The Bible says people like this are observing the letter of the law but not the spirit. However, being a Christian means more than observing the letter of the law. Moral purity means more than just abstaining from intercourse.

2. What does it mean to defraud someone? (1 point)
    To defraud means to arouse sexual desires in another which cannot be righteously fulfilled.

3. Why does God allow young people such strong sexual desires and then commands them to abstain from sex until marriage? (2 points)
    The temptations you face as a teenager will still be with you as an adult. Learning self-control during this difficult time will help you face the same temptations as an adult. Furthermore, people used to marry at a much younger age when lifestyles and customs were different from today.

4. List 4 <u>reasons</u> Josh McDowell gives <u>for waiting</u> until marriage for sexual involvement. (4 points)
    - *Protects from unplanned pregnancy and provides a healthy atmosphere for child-rearing.*
    - *Protects from sexually transmitted diseases and provides for peace of mind.*
    - *Protects from sexual insecurity and provides for truth.*
    - *Protects from emotional distress and provides for true intimacy.*

5. List 5 ways Josh McDowell gives for how to wait until marriage for sexual involvement. (5 points)
    - *Set standards beforehand and share these standards with your dates.*
    - *Be accountable to your parents or to another person regarding your dating behavior.*
    - *Let your lifestyle show through conversation, body language and clothes.*
    - *Know yourself and be your own person.*
    - *Choose companions carefully: hang around people with the same values.*
    - *Seek others' wisdom: get counsel or advice when you are involved in a friendship.*

6. A friend of yours says she is pregnant. She comes to you for help. She is considering an abortion. What do you tell her? (3 points)

    Give her acceptance and love and not condemnation. Tell her that God loves her and her family will too. Tell her you will go with her to tell her parents or guardian. Also explain the options to having an abortion. She can give the baby to a good, Christian home through adoption, she could raise the child alone or she could marry the father. Be realistic about the way her life would change if she raised the child alone. Furthermore, most teen fathers are not committed to the relationship when a girl becomes pregnant. The most important thing is to encourage her to seek help. Give her the name and number of a Crisis Pregnancy Center and go with her to a counselor.

7. Why do many teens experiment with tobacco? What advice would you give a friend who began to smoke and use chewing tobacco? (3 points)

    Many teens experiment because of peer pressure. There are many harmful effects of using tobacco:

    - *Stains your teeth and makes your clothes smell.*
    - *Can cause serious illnesses and diseases.*
    - *It is expensive.*
    - *It is often banned in public places.*
    - *Dulls your sense of smell and taste.*
    - *Can become addictive.*
    - *It is not "cool" anymore.*
    - *Harmful to your brain, mouth, larynx, skin, lungs, heart, digestive system, bladder and legs.*

8. Why do some teenagers choose to drink alcohol? What would you say to a friend who was beginning to drink alcohol? (3 points)

Teenagers drink mostly because of peer pressure, some drink to avoid their problems, and many think it is "cool" to drink. Tell your friend:

- *Drinking can be habit forming.*
- *Alcohol negatively affects the body: the brain, skin, liver, heart and bloodstream, kidneys, digestive system, and reproductive system.*
- *Drinking is not "cool."*
- *Drinking does not take away your problems, it only creates more for you.*

9. You are at a party and a friend hands you a glass of alcohol. Give two things you can say to your friend to tell him you do not want it. (2 points)
    - *"No, I don't drink."*
    - *"If you were my friend you would not ask me if I wanted this."*
    - *"I am going now, do you want to come."*

TOTAL HEALTH

CHAPTER 13: TEST

Unit 3: Social Health

KEY

100 points

MATCHING (2 points each): For each item on the left column, find the appropriate answer on the right column. Place the letter of the correct answer in the space provided at the left of each item. Each answer may be used only once.

1. _F_ Puberty
2. _G_ Abortion
3. _E_ Defraud
4. _K_ Nicotine
5. _D_ Tar
6. _I_ Carbon Monoxide
7. _H_ Emphysema
8. _B_ Drugs
9. _C_ Medicines
10. _O_ Stimulants
11. _N_ Addiction
12. _M_ Depressants
13. _J_ Fetal Alcohol Syndrome
14. _A_ Alcoholism

A. Habitual, compulsive, long-term drinking.
B. Chemical substance that alters organ function.
C. Meant to cure or prevent diseases.
D. Main cause of lung cancer; thick, dark, liquid.
E. Arouse sexual desires that can't be fulfilled.
F. Stage of growth and development at which males and females are able to reproduce.
G. Medically induced termination of pregnancy.
H. Small air sacs called alveoli are damaged or destroyed.
I. Produced when tobacco burns.
J. Causes abnormal limb development, retardation, cleft palate, heart disease.
K. Acts like a tranquilizer and causes addiction to tobacco.
L. Never drive with someone who has been drinking.
M. Slow down body's functions and reactions.
N. A physical or mental need for a substance.
O. Speed up the body's functions: can become addictive.

Copyright © 1995 Susan Boe

Chapter Thirteen, Test Key, page 2 of 5

SHORT ANSWER AND FILL IN THE BLANK: Answer the following questions (note the points given to each question).

15. How is the human race unlike any other living being? (3 points)
    God has given humans volumes of common sense and wisdom. People have the ability to know where they came from, know where they want to go, how they want to live and what they want to do. People also have the capacity to know right from wrong.

16. How can the "right now" mentality be dangerous? (3 points)
    Society is a "right now" society. You don't always know the long-term results of your decisions. Furthermore, the benefits of making right choices are not always instantaneous. This can be a dangerous attitude because you may do things that will negatively affect your life because you do not see the consequences right away. Right choices often require waiting for long-term results.

17. Why does God place boundaries in your life? (2 points)
    God places boundaries in your life not to see you fail or to have you be unhappy, but to protect you.

18. Why does God allow young people such strong sexual desires and then commands them to abstain from sex until marriage? (3 points)
    The temptations you face as a teenager will still be with you as an adult. Learning self-control during this difficult time will help you face the same temptations as an adult. Furthermore, people use to marry at a much younger age when lifestyles and customs were different than today.

19. How many times does it take to use an illegal drug before it might kill you? (1 point)
    Once.

20. Explain the meaning of the phrase, "abstinence is not the only goal." (3 points)
    Many young people go "too far" without "going all the way." That is, they engage in sexual activity but do not have intercourse. The Bible says people like this are observing the letter of the law but not the spirit. However, being a Christian means more than observing the letter of the law. Moral purity means more than just abstaining from intercourse.

21. What is the main reason why teens experiment with alcohol, tobacco, and drugs? (2 points)
    Peer pressure.

22. List 4 harmful effects of the use of tobacco (smoking or chewing). (4 points)
    - *Stains your teeth and makes your clothes smell.*
    - *Can cause serious illnesses and diseases.*
    - *It is expensive.*
    - *It is often banned in public places.*
    - *Dulls your sense of smell and taste.*
    - *Can become addictive.*
    - *It is not "cool" anymore.*
    - *Harmful to your brain, mouth, larynx, skin, lungs, heart, digestive system, bladder and legs.*

23. What would you say to a friend who was beginning to drink alcohol? (4 points)
    Teenagers drink mostly because of peer pressure, some drink to avoid their problems, and many think it is "cool" to drink. Tell your friend:

    - *Drinking can be habit forming.*
    - *Alcohol negatively affects the body: the brain, skin, liver, heart and bloodstream, kidneys, digestive system, and reproductive system.*
    - *Drinking is not "cool."*
    - *Drinking does not take away your problems, it only creates more for you.*

24. What is the most precious gift you can give your future mate? (2 points)
    Your virginity is the most precious gift.

25. **ESSAY** (20 points): Maturity is not only physical but emotional, social and spiritual. Write an essay entitled: "What it means to be mature."

Include in your answer:
- The cause of emotional highs and lows. (2 points)
- 8 signs of maturity (not physical maturity). (8 points)
- What is social maturity? (2 points)
- What aspect of maturity should concern you the most? Why? (4 points)
- Why does God place boundaries in your life? (2 points)
- How does a teen's curiosity show his level of maturity? (2 points)

- *The cause of emotional highs and lows are: hormonal changes.*

- *Signs of maturity:*
  - *Has self-control.*
  - *Recognizes godly values: makes good judgments.*
  - *Recognizes the importance of setting goals.*
  - *Stands up for what is right even when persecuted.*
  - *Assume responsibility for actions.*
  - *Avoids compromising situations.*
  - *Avoids being judgmental or critical of others.*
  - *Is able to be trusted.*
  - *Respects others: forms mature relationships.*
  - *Has more concern for others: not so self-centered.*

- *Social maturity is the ability a person has to relate to others in a proper way. Respect.*

- *Spiritual maturity is the maturity that you should be concerned the most about because you are investing in an eternal relationship with God.*

- *God places boundaries in your life to protect you.*

- *Curiosity is normal, but it is how you deal with it that shows your level of maturity. It is what you allow yourself to think about and investigate that can cause you problems.*

26. **ESSAY** (20 points): You and a friend are talking late one night. Your friend says he/she is feeling pressured to engage in sexual activity. He/she wants to know what you think about sex before marriage and "how far is too far" in the area of physical involvement. Explain to your friend:
- Why you feel waiting until marriage is important. (5 points)
- Tell your friend how he/she can wait until marriage. (5 points)
- Explain to your friend why "abstinence is not the only goal." (5 points)
- Explain to your friend why this is such a big decision in his/her life. (5 points)

- *Waiting until marriage is important because:*
  - *Protects from unplanned pregnancy and provides a healthy atmosphere for child-rearing.*
  - *Protects from sexually transmitted diseases and provides for peace of mind.*
  - *Protects from sexual insecurity and provides for truth.*
  - *Protects from emotional distress and provides for true intimacy.*

- *How can he/she wait:*
  - *Set standards beforehand and share these standards with your dates.*
  - *Be accountable to your parents or to another person regarding your dating behavior.*
  - *Let your lifestyle show through conversation, body language and clothes.*
  - *Know yourself and be your own person.*
  - *Choose companions carefully: hang around people with the same values.*
  - *Seek others' wisdom: get counsel or advice when you are involved in a friendship.*

- *Abstinence is not the only goal:*
  Many young people go "too far" without "going all the way." That is, they engage in sexual activity but do not have intercourse. The Bible says people like this are observing the letter of the law but not the spirit. However, being a Christian means more than observing the letter of the law. Moral purity means more than just abstaining from intercourse.

- *It is such a big decision because:*
  You don't always know the consequences of your actions until later. Although it may seem difficult to wait now, the rewards are worth it.

TOTAL HEALTH

CHAPTER 14: QUIZ A

Unit 3: Social Health

KEY

Sections: 14-1, 14-2
25 points

SHORT ANSWER: Answer the following questions (note the points given to each question).

1. Why is dating not always fun? (2 points)
    There is a certain social pressure that comes with dating. It can make friendships uncomfortable. It also takes up more of your time and mental and emotional energy when you could be spending time on school and other activities.

2. What 3 suggestions can you make when making your decision about dating? (3 points)
    1. Group date.
    2. Make specific plans.
    3. Be creative.

3. Explain the following diagram as it relates to relationships with the opposite sex. Fill in the numbered blanks in the diagram. (6 points)

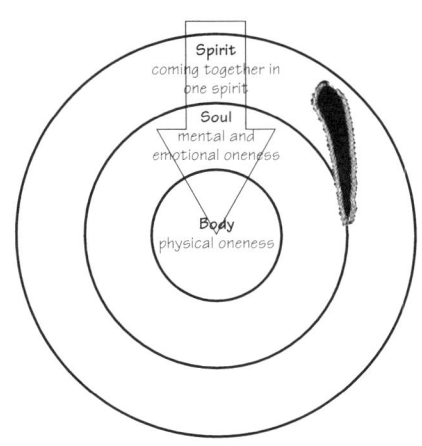

    Possible answer may include:
    God's order for successful relationships with the opposite sex is to take the time in groups to get to know people spiritually and emotionally. Even if this seems difficult and against what "everyone" else is doing, it is worth the effort. Having feelings toward a person of the opposite sex is normal, it is how you handle these feelings that is important. "Do not use the world's way to relate or you will have the world's result" (Wendell Smith). The physical connection between two people is the last type of "oneness" that should be experienced and it is to be saved for marriage.

4. Explain the difference between *Agape* love and *Eros* love. (3 points)

   Agape love is the most common word of all forms of love in the New Testament. Expresses love from the Father to the Son, God to man, and man to God and man to his neighbor. Jesus' whole life was Agape love in action. Agape is selfless.

   Eros love is the more natural form of love, liking to do things that are pleasant. Eros is more selfish.

5. List 3 reasons for marriage as Dennis Rainey states in his book *Staying Close*. (3 points)
   - *To mirror God's image.*
   - *To multiply a godly heritage.*
   - *To manage God's realm.*
   - *To mutually complete one another.*
   - *To model Christ's relationship to the church.*

6. List and explain the 4 myths of marriage. (4 points)

   1. "Marriage is just not worth it."
   Young people grow up thinking that marriage hurts and is not worth the effort since it will probably end in divorce.

   2. "But I thought it would be different."
   Many people enter into marriage with expectations that cannot be fulfilled.

   3. "If it doesn't work out, I will just get a divorce."
   Divorce is not the answer to a troubled marriage. When you enter marriage with this in mind, you have already set yourself up for problems.

   4. "I have it all planned out."
   God doesn't frown on making plans and having goals and dreams, but planning things you have no control over can leave you open for great disappointments.

7. Explain how you can prepare yourself for the commitment of marriage. (2 points)
   - *Grow in your relationship to the Lord*
   - *Develop the character qualities that will make you the best marriage partner you can be.*

8. What is the key to life? (2 points)

   The key to life is not marriage but your relationship to God.

TOTAL HEALTH   CHAPTER 14: QUIZ B

Unit: 3 Social Health

KEY

Sections: 14-3, 14-4
25 points

FILL IN THE BLANK AND SHORT ANSWER: Answer the following questions (note the points given to each question).

1. Teenagers are not ready to be parents. Give 3 reasons why this is true. (3 points)
   1. *Most teens do not have the money or resources to provide what a child needs.*
   2. *During your teens you are still learning who you are and what you want to do in life.*
   3. *Having a child when you are not emotionally ready also is bad for you as well as for the child.*

2. List 4 helpful hints to getting along with your family. (4 points)
   - *Avoid serious conversations when you know you are already upset.*
   - *Communicate clearly what you feel before you lose your temper.*
   - *Really listen when the other person is sharing.*
   - *Avoid using phrases like "you never...," or "you always..."*
   - *Use other opportunities to build up your family members.*
   - *Use phrases like, "this makes me feel...."*
   - *Be honest; that means, share how you really feel.*
   - *Pray for the person you are having a hard time with.*
   - *Pick a time to sit down and talk.*
   - *Remember to say, "I am sorry." and "please forgive me."*
   - *Avoid the temptation to "get back" at the person.*
   - *Make time to communicate with your parents.*

3. Nothing is as easy as *talking,* nothing is as difficult as *communicating.* (2 points)

4. List 4 positive ways you should treat the elderly. (4 points).
   1. *Make allowances for their age and mobility.*
   2. *Seek their advice.*
   3. *React enthusiastically to their plans or thoughts.*
   4. *Involve them in your activities.*
   5. *Tell them they are important.*

Copyright © 1995 Susan Boe

5. List 3 physical signs of aging. (3 points)
    1. *Skin and hair: gradual loss of elastic tissue in the skin. And hair loss.*
    2. *Skeleton and muscles: bones and joints become stiffer. Muscles become weaker.*
    3. *Heart and circulation: the heart has to work harder. Blood pressure may rise.*
    4. *Lungs: breathing ability is reduced.*
    5. *Abdominal organs: lose their efficiency.*
    6. *Senses: weakening of the senses. Especially hearing and seeing.*

6. What is Alzheimer's disease? (1 point)
    A form of mental slow down.

7. List 3 of the 5 common reactions to experiencing a loss. (3 points)
    1. *Shock*
    2. *Anger*
    3. *Longing*
    4. *Depression*
    5. *Going on*

8. Give 3 ways to help someone cope with a loss. (3 points)
    1. *Encourage them to express their feelings.*
    2. *Respect your friend's right to feeling sad or depressed.*
    3. *Give them the time they need to "move on."*
    4. *Help them to remember the good things about their loved one.*

9. A friend of yours fears death and dying. What can you tell her to help her cope with her feelings? (2 points)
    Some people fear how they will die and others fear what will happen after they die. If you know the Lord before you die you can be assured there is spiritual life after physical death. A better place awaits you than life here on earth.

TOTAL HEALTH

CHAPTER 14: TEST

Unit 3: Social Health

KEY

100 points

FILL IN THE BLANK AND SHORT ANSWER: Answer the following questions (note the points given to each question).

1. Explain the four levels of friendships in the following pryamid as it relates to your friendship with the opposite sex. Fill-in the appropriate answers where needed. (4 points)

    The number of friends naturally decreases as you go up the pyramid levels. The first level is based on casual contacts, the second level based on common interests and activities, the third level is based on mutual goals and the fourth level is based on commitment to the development of each other's character. The close and intimate levels of friendship are reserved for a person with whom you are considering marriage.

    Pyramid labels:
    - Four: Intimate Level — Based on commitment to the development of each other's character
    - Three: Close — Based on mutual life goals
    - Two: Casual — Based on common interests and activities
    - One: Acquaintance — Based on casual contacts

2. Dating is not always fun. Why is this true? (2 points)

    There is a certain social pressure that comes with dating. It can make friendships uncomfortable. It also takes up more of your time and mental and emotional energy when you could be spending time on school and other activities.

3. What 3 suggestions can you make when making your decision about dating? (3 points)

    1. Group date.
    2. Make specific plans.
    3. Be creative

4. Explain the following diagram as it relates to relationships with the opposite sex. Fill in the appropriate blanks in the diagram. (6 points)

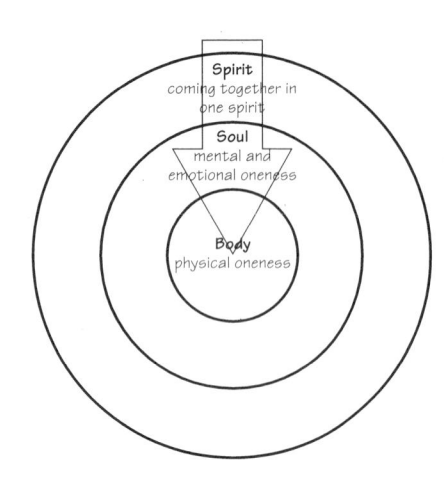

Diagram labels:
- Spirit — coming together in one spirit
- Soul — mental and emotional oneness
- Body — physical oneness

Possible answer may include:
God's order for successful relationships with the opposite sex is to take the time in groups to get to know people spiritually and emotionally. Even if this seems difficult and against what "everyone" else is doing, it is worth the effort. Having feelings toward a person of the opposite sex is normal, it is how you handle these feelings that is important. "Do not use the world's way to relate or you will have the world's result" (Wendell Smith). The physical connection between two people is the last type of "oneness" that should be experienced and it is to be saved for marriage.

5. Why is it a good idea to go on group dates? (3 points)

   Group dating allows you to get to know people of the opposite sex without the social pressures that come with being alone on a date. You do not have that awkward feeling of being alone, not knowing what to say or do. Also being able to watch your friends in different situations helps you get to know them.

6. What is meant by the phrase, "sex and love are not synonymous"? (3 points)

   They are two separate concepts. Sex is an act performed by two people committed to loving each other for life, while love, in varying degrees, can be felt by anyone. Love is not an act; love is a commitment.

7. Respond to the following "lines" concerning pressure to be sexually active. (4 points)

   Line 1: "Everybody's doing it."
   Reply: *That's great. Then I guess you won't have any problem finding someone else.*

   Line 2: "If you love me, you'll have sex with me."
   Reply: *If you love me, you'll respect my feelings and not push me into doing something I'm not ready for.*

   Line 3: "We had sex once before, so what's the problem now?"
   Reply: *I have a right to change my mind. I've decided to wait.*

   Line 4: "Don't you want to try it to see what it is like?"
   Reply: *What is this? Some kind of commercial? Try it; you'll like it! I do plan to try it ...with my husband (wife).*

8. List and explain the 4 myths of marriage. (4 points)
   1. *"Marriage is just not worth it."*
      Young people grow up thinking that marriage hurts and is not worth the effort since it will probably end in divorce.

   2. *"But I thought it would be different."*
      Many people enter into marriage with expectations that cannot be fulfilled.

   3. *"If it doesn't work out, I will just get a divorce."*
      Divorce is not the answer to a troubled marriage. When you enter marriage with this in mind, you have already set yourself up for problems.

   4. *"I have it all planned out."*
      God doesn't frown on making plans and having goals and dreams, but planning things you have no control over can leave you open for great disappointments.

9. List 5 reasons for marriage as Dennis Rainey states in his book *Staying Close*. (5 points)
   - *To mirror God's image.*
   - *To multiply a godly heritage.*
   - *To manage God's realm.*
   - *To mutually complete one another.*
   - *To model Christ's relationship to the church.*

10. What is the key to life? (3 points)
    The key to life is not marriage but your relationship to God.

11. Give 3 reasons why teenagers are not ready to be parents. (3 points)
    1. *Most teens do not have the money or resources to provide what a child needs.*
    2. *During your teens you are still learning who you are and what you want to do in life.*
    3. *Having a child when you are not emotionally ready also is bad for you as well as for the child.*

12. List 4 positive ways you should treat the elderly. (4 points)
    1. *Make allowances for their age and mobility.*
    2. *Seek their advice.*
    3. *React enthusiastically to their plans or thoughts.*
    4. *Involve them in your activities.*
    5. *Tell them they are important.*

13. List 3 physical signs of aging. (3 points)
    1. *Skin and hair: gradual loss of elastic tissue in the skin. And hair loss.*
    2. *Skeleton and muscles: bones and joints become stiffer. Muscles become weaker.*
    3. *Heart and circulation: the heart has to work harder. Blood pressure may rise.*
    4. *Lungs: breathing ability is reduced.*
    5. *Abdominal organs: lose their efficiency.*
    6. *Senses: weakening of the senses. Especially hearing and seeing.*

14. Nothing is as easy as _talking,_ nothing is as difficult as _communicating._ (2 points)

15. What is Alzheimer's disease? (1 point)
    A form of mental slow down.

16. **ESSAY** (25 points): Write an essay entitled:

    "Kingdom relationships vs. the culture's way of dating."

Summarize the following chart in your essay.

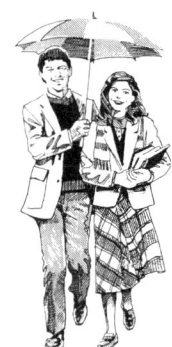

Answer: Make sure the student brings in each of the four points from the chart and compares kingdom relationships with culture's way of relating. Grade on style, clarity and completeness of answer. The chart gives the information so the student only needs to organize their thoughts and use proper grammar and punctuation.

	God's Ways of "Kingdom Relationships" God-centered relationships		Culture's Way of "Dating": Self-centered relationships
Basis:	Wholesome attraction Commitment to God Friendship	Basis:	Natural attraction Feelings, desires
Goal:	Mutual edification and fulfillment of God's will	Goal:	Mutual gratification and fulfillment of self-will
Qualities:	Giving attitude Absolute moral standards Focus on Spirit and Soul Taking time to get to know each other Relationship inclusive of the Body of Christ	Qualities:	Receiving attitude No absolutes, no standards Focus on Body and Soul Moving quickly to take advantage of each other Relationship exclusive and possessive
Results:	Stronger relationship to the Lord and others Healthy self-image Character development for better Greater motivation Increased fulfillment Good example to others Peace, joy and abundant life	Results:	Weakened relationships with God and others Unhealthy self-image Character change for worse Draining of motivation Decreased fulfillment Influence others to sin Confusion, strife and heartache Emptiness and sorrow

17. **ESSAY** (25 points each): Write an essay on <u>one</u> of the following topics:

A. How to handle conflicts in my family
   - 10 helpful hints to getting along. (10 points)
   - Examples of personal situations you experience in your family. (5 points)
   - What is the main reason people get upset at one another in the family with no apparent reason? (5 points)
   - If you cannot talk to someone in your family about the conflicts, who can you turn to for help? (5 points)

   Answers to A:
   - *Helpful hints to getting along with your family:*
     - *Avoid serious conversations when you know you are already upset.*
     - *Communicate clearly what you feel before you lose your temper.*
     - *Really listen when the other person is sharing.*
     - *Avoid using phrases like "you never...," or "you always..."*
     - *Use other opportunities to build up your family members.*
     - *Use phrases like, "this makes me feel...."*
     - *Be honest; that means, share how you really feel.*
     - *Pray for the person you are having a hard time with.*
     - *Pick a time to sit down and talk.*
     - *Remember to say, "I am sorry" and "please forgive me."*
     - *Avoid the temptation to "get back" at the person.*
     - *Make time to communicate with your parents.*

   - *People get upset for no apparent reason because of the roller-coaster ride of emotions they are experiencing.*

   - *You can turn to an adult you trust. Your pastor, parent of a friend, teacher or counselor at school.*

B. Understanding grief
   - The defintion of grief. (5 points)
   - What are the 5 common reactions to experiencing loss. (5 points)
   - Give 4 ways to help someone cope with a loss. (4 points)
   - What to say to someone who is fearful of death. (5 points)
   - What can you say to someone who has experienced a loss? (5 points)
   - A personal example of you or someone you know who experienced grief and how you (they) handled it. If you don't have one, explain how you feel when you think about losing someone you love. (1 point)

Answers to B:

- *The definition of grief is: all the feelings of sorrow and deep distress over a death of a loved one.*

- *5 common reactions: Shock, anger, longing, depression and going on.*

- *Ways to help someone cope:*
    - *Encourage them to express their feelings.*
    - *Respect their right to feeling sad or depressed.*
    - *Give them the time they need to "move on."*
    - *Help them to remember the good things about their loved one.*

- *One who is fearful of death: "If you know the Lord, physical death means spiritual life.*

- *It is better to say nothing to a person who just experienced a loss. Do not try to counsel or answer their question of why it happened. Just be with the person and be a friend.*

TOTAL HEALTH

CHAPTER 15: QUIZ A

Unit 4: Spiritual Health

KEY

Section: 15-1
25 points

FILL IN THE BLANK AND SHORT ANSWER: Answer the following questions (note the points given to each question).

1. Explain the meaning of spiritual atrophy. (2 points)
   Think of yourself as a spiritual athlete. you have spiritual muscles that must be exercised in order to keep them fit. If you do not pay attention to your spiritual muscles, you will atrophy and will find yourself spiritually weak and unprepared for spiritual activity.

2. What are 5 signs of spiritual atrophy? (5 points)
   - *Have you been feeling like God is far away?*
   - *Have you been struggling with temptation and sin lately?*
   - *Have you had difficulty getting along with someone?*
   - *Have you had little desire to read the Bible?*
   - *Have you had little desire to attend church or church activities?*

3. The __*Bible*__ is the training manual for spiritual fitness. (1 point)
4. __*Biblical*__ meditation will transform your life by transforming your __*thoughts*__ and your __*heart.*__ (3 points)
5. List the 5 basic keys to spiritual training. (5 points)
   - *Bible reading and meditation on the Word of God.*
   - *Private prayer times and being quiet in His presence.*
   - *Fellowshipping with other believers; church and other activities.*
   - *GIGO: God in— God out: serving and telling others about God.*
   - *Praise and worship.*

6. What does it mean to meditate on the Bible? (1 point)
   To reflect on and think about what you have read.

7. What would you tell a friend who said, "I don't want to pray because I have sinned." (2 points)

   God is faithful to forgive you of your mistakes if you ask Him. You have a choice, you can continue to be troubled by it or you can make things right with God and others. Spiritual breathing is exhaling by confessing the sin and then inhaling God's forgiveness.

8. What would you tell a friend who said, "I don't *feel* like praying." (2 points)

   Feelings are hard to control. Feeling tired, depressed, anxious etc., are real feelings that can keep you from praying. If you come to your prayer time each day and ignore your feelings, you will reap the benefits of spending time with God. Tell God how you feel and He will help you.

9. Explain the following format for praying. (4 points)

   A *Adoration: to worship and honor God for who He is.*

   C *Confession: to ask God for forgiveness for thoughts, actions, behaviors that have not pleased Him.*

   T *Thanksgiving: to give thanks to God for all He has done for you.*

   S *Supplication: to bring concerns, worries and petitions before Him. To ask for guidance and provision for yourself and for others.*

TOTAL HEALTH — CHAPTER 15: QUIZ B

Unit 4: Spiritual Health

KEY

Section: 15-2
25 points

SHORT ANSWER: Answer the following questions (note the points given to each question).

1. What is meant by the phrase, "Christianity is not a do-it-yourself project?" (3 points)
   You are not left to fight this battle alone. If you have God in your heart, then you also have the power of the Holy Spirit. You have the power of Christ in you to help you live a life that is pleasing to Him.

2. What is to be in the Control Tower of your life? (2 points)
   The Word of God.

3. What are the 5 keys to consistent Christian living? (5 points)
   - *Renewing the mind.*
   - *Growing in Christian virtues.*
   - *Discipline.*
   - *Perseverance.*
   - *Have a vision for your life.*

4. What are five practical steps to renewing your mind? (5 points)
   - *Study, meditate and memorize the Word of God.*
   - *Spend time in prayer.*
   - *Listen to edifying music.*
   - *Read edifying material.*
   - *Discipline your tongue to only speak what is edifying.*

5. What things might keep teenagers from living a consistent Christian life? (3 points)
   - *Peer pressure.*
   - *Yielding to temptation.*
   - *Other answers may be appropriate.*

6. What does the phrase mean, "Growth in all areas of the Christian life is progressive." (2 points)

It is worked out over a period of time and the growth is never finished. You will never "arrive" at a place where you can quit pursuing the things of God.

7. What role does discipline have in living a consistent Christian life? (3 points)

Just as training for a sport takes discipline, so does your Christian life. You must apply yourself to certain skills and discipline yourself to practice these skills. You will learn how to pray, how to develop godly character, how to praise Him and how to read the Bible. It is not always easy, but the rewards are great.

8. What does living a consistent Christian life mean? (2 points)

Having a solid and stable lifestyle pleasing to God.

TOTAL HEALTH

CHAPTER 15: TEST

Unit 4: Spiritual Health

KEY

100 points

SHORT ANSWER: Answer the following questions (note the points given to each question).

1. Explain the meaning of spiritual atrophy. (2 points)
    Think of yourself as a spiritual athlete. You have spiritual muscles that must be exercised in order to keep them fit. If you do not pay attention to your spiritual muscles, you will atrophy and will find yourself spiritually weak and unprepared for spiritual activity.

2. What are 5 signs of spiritual atrophy? (5 points)
    - *Have you been feeling like God is far away?*
    - *Have you been struggling with temptation and sin lately?*
    - *Have you had difficulty getting along with someone?*
    - *Have you had little desire to read the Bible?*
    - *Have you had little desire to attend church or church activities?*

3. List the 5 basic keys to spiritual training. (5 points)
    - *Bible reading and meditation on the Word of God.*
    - *Private prayer times and being quiet in His presence.*
    - *Fellowshipping with other believers; church and other activities.*
    - *GIGO: God in— God out: serving and telling others about God.*
    - *Praise and worship.*

4. What is the meaning of righteousness? What is *training in righteousness*? (4 points)
    Righteousness is conformity to the law, mind and will of God. Training in righteousness is a lifestyle, not a temporary achievement. It is learning how to conform to God's law, mind and His will.

5. What is the training manual for spiritual fitness? (2 points)
    The Bible.

6. How will meditating on the Bible transform you life? (2 points)
    By transforming your thoughts and your heart.

7. What are the 6 practical steps to Bible reading? (6 points)
    1. *Have your own Bible.*
    2. *Make a definite reading program.*
    3. *Choose a specific time of day.*
    4. *Pray, ask God to help you as you read.*
    5. *Mark your Bible or take notes in a notebook.*
    6. *Put the Bible to memory. Choose scriptures that encourage you and memorize them.*

8. Where does the desire to read the Bible or to pray come from? (2 points)
    God.

9. What would you tell a friend who asked, "Why should I pray?" (4 points)
    - *Prayer gives you strength to face the challenges of life.*
    - *Prayer causes you to see yourself as you truly are; in deep need for God.*
    - *Prayer helps you to be more kind and loving to others.*
    - *Prayer can bring health and healing to your body and mind.*
    - *Prayer causes you to become more like Christ.*

10. What would you tell a friend who said, "But I don't have time to pray." (4 points)
    If you really want to do something you will fit it in your schedule. Take five minutes to pray in the morning before you get ready for school. It might seem like an effort, but those five minutes will increase because you want to spend more time with God.

11. Explain the following format for praying. (4 points)
    A *Adoration: to worship and honor God for who He is.*

    C *Confession: to ask God for forgiveness for thoughts, actions, behaviors that have not pleased Him.*

    T *Thanksgiving: to give thanks to God for all He has done for you.*

    S *Supplication: to bring concerns, worries and petitions before Him. To ask for guidance and provision for yourself and for others.*

12. What is to be in the Control Tower of your life? (2 points)
    The Word of God.

13. What is meant by spiritual breathing? (4 points)
    In order to stay physically healthy we must exhale to cleanse the carbon dioxide from the air and then inhale to replenish the oxygen. In the same way Christians need to "breathe spiritually" to stay spiritually healthy. The moment the Holy Spirit convicts us of sin, we should "exhale" by confessing that sin to God....After exhaling the impure, we can "inhale" the pure....and receive God's forgiveness.

14. What does it mean to "pray the Word of God?" Why is it important to do this? (4 points)
    When you speak the Bible out loud in prayer you know God hears you because it is God's will written for you. Speaking the Word of God will increase your faith in all that God can do.

15. What is meant by the phrase, "Christianity is not a do-it-yourself project." (3 points)
    You are not left to fight this battle alone. If you have God in your heart, then you also have the power of the Holy Spirit. You have the power of Christ in you to help you live a life that is pleasing to Him.

16. What things might keep teenagers from living a consistent Christian life? (3 points)
    - *Peer pressure.*
    - *Yielding to temptation.*
    - *Other answers may be appropriate.*

17. What role does discipline have in living a consistent Christian life? (4 points)
    Just as training for a sport takes discipline, so does your Christian life. You must apply yourself to certain skills and discipline yourself to practice these skills. You will learn how to pray, how to develop godly character, how to praise Him and how to read the Bible. It is not always easy, but the rewards are great.

18. **ESSAY** (20 points)
You are asked to speak at a youth gathering. The title of your message is:

"How to live a consistent Christian life."

Include in your message:
- The 5 keys to consistent Christian living. (5 points)
- Explain each key to consistent Christian living. (5 points)
- 5 Specific examples that teens may struggle with in their Christian walk and how to deal with them. (10 points)

Answer to question 18:
- *Keys to consistent living:*
    1. *Renewing your mind.*
    2. *Growing in Christian virtues.*
    3. *Discipline.*
    4. *Perseverance.*
    5. *Have a vision for your life.*

19. **ESSAY** (20 points)
You are asked to speak at your youth group. The title of your message is:

"Getting off the fence."

Include in your message:
- What is a spiritual fence? (5 points)
- What to do if you lack the desire to serve God. (5 points)
- 5 Specific examples that may keep teens riding the spiritual fence and how to deal with them. (10 points)

Possible answer may include:
> *Note: the student's answer should be "up beat" and positive because they are to be talking to a youth group on the subject. It should be motivational and insightful.*
- *A spiritual fence is holding the position of indecision trying to decide whether to live a life that is pleasing to God or pleasing to self. Serve Him totally.*
- *If a person lacks the desire to serve God he needs to pray to God to ask Him to give him more of a desire to desire more of Him. Also, if there are things hindering that person from godly things such as the wrong influences or sinful behavior then the person needs to deal with those things. Listen to God and then respond.*
- *5 examples: peer pressure, desire to conform, rebellious toward authority, lacking trust in God, family problems, negative friendships, sinful lifestyle, etc.*

TOTAL HEALTH CHAPTER 16: QUIZ A

Unit 4: Spiritual Health

KEY

Section: 16-1
25 points

FILL IN THE BLANK AND SHORT ANSWER: Answer the following questions (note the points given to each question).

1. Explain the following verse as it relates to teenagers: "Without a vision the people perish." Proverbs 29:18 (3 points)
    With your eyes on a vision (or motivating cause) for your life, the distractions that can hinder you are reduced. Each believer has a purpose for living, a purpose beyond living for yourself. Having a vision for your life.

2. Seeking a __purpose__ for living means seeking the __creator__ of that purpose. (2 points)

3. Who is the source of the vision for your life? (2 points)
    God.

4. Explain why it is important not to get "hung-up" on issues that can distract you from the purposes of God. What are some examples of these issues that might distract teenagers from the purposes of God? (3 points)
    Some issues can distract teens away from what God wants to do in their lives. Examples are: Fashion, hairstyles, popularity, etc.

5. Explain the following: "In the same way that a wall is built, stone by stone, you find and walk out your destiny in God a little at a time." (5 points)
    Each brick, when placed in just the right place at the right time, provides extra strength to the structure. As you work to build your life by placing the right principles and commandments together, you will fashion a strong fortress that can withstand opposition. (Luke 16:10, He who is faithful in little, is faithful in much). As you walk out the basic Christian walk, being faithful with what God is doing now, you will find yourself walking in the very purpose God has for your life.

6. What is meant by the term Destiny? (3 points)

   Something that is to happen to a particular person or thing. The predetermined course of events.

7. Your _goal_ in life is not to decide what _you_ want to do, but to discover what _He_ destined you to do! (3 points)

8. Explain the connection between the words **pleasure** and **will** as they are used in the two versions of Revelation 4:11. How does this relate to God's vision for your life? (4 points)

   "You are worthy, O Lord, To receive glory and honor and power. For You created all thing, And by Your **will** they exist and were created." Revelation 4:11 (NKJ)

   "Thou are worthy, O Lord, to receive glory and honor and power: for thou hast created all things, and for thy **pleasure** they are and were created." Revelation 4:11 (KJV)

   God chose to create you for a specific purpose. His will (desire) for you is that you find His purpose, walk it out in your lifetime, and ultimately reach the potential God has planned for you. This gives Him great pleasure!

TOTAL HEALTH

CHAPTER 16: QUIZ B

Unit 4: Spiritual Health

KEY

Sections: 16-2, 16-3
25 points

FILL IN THE BLANK AND SHORT ANSWER: Answer the following questions (note the points given to each question).

1. Why is it important not to "borrow trouble?" (5 points)

    It is important not to worry about things that you don't even know will come to pass. Bill Meyer and Dan Zandra say this: We spend so much time thinking about how we might lose, that we forget to think about how we might win. Instead of thinking about how well we're going to do, we spend all our practice time thinking up imaginary disasters for ourselves.

    People need to concentrate on the promises of God. You are on a winning team. There is no way you can lose if you stay on His team. Train yourself, speaking out the promises of God. Be "God-Focused."

2. What is the meaning of the *cross* in the life of a Christian? (3 points)

    The cross in the life of a Christian is the crossing of two wills, yours and God's.

3. What are 4 hindrances to reaching your destiny? Of these 4 hindrances what is the strongest according to James Dobson? (5 points)
    - *Lack of motivation.*
    - *Laziness.*
    - *Rebellious attitudes.*
    - *Lack of discipline: learn to discipline the flesh, this being the strongest hindrance to reaching your potential.*

4. The greatest deterrent to __*sin*__ is not religious rules, but __*vision.*__ (2 points)

5. Why do shortcuts usually lead away from growth, not toward it? (3 points)

    There is something in everyone that wants instant results, ultimately avoiding the process of learning. God does not promise that you can avoid or skip over the trials. He does, however, promise to be with you as you walk through them.

Chapter Sixteen, Quiz B Key, page 2 of 2

6. Explain the following verse of scripture. (2 points)

"And let us not grow weary while doing good, for in due season we shall reap if we do not lose heart." Galatians 6:9

God knows the struggles you face and that you can become spiritually exhausted from trying to do the "right" thing. You will receive more from God by remaining steadfast.

7. What is the answer to weariness of spirit? (2 points)
The answer is to wait on the Lord. Wait with patience, anticipation and with humility in His presence.

8. What is your ultimate inheritance in heaven? (1 point)
To enjoy Jesus Christ forever.

9. How is a person assured of having a place in the Father's house? Does this assurance make your life on earth easier? Why or why not? (2 points)
Salvation through Jesus Christ as your personal Lord and Saviour.

TOTAL HEALTH

CHAPTER 16: TEST

Unit 4: Spiritual Health

KEY

100 points

FILL IN THE BLANK AND SHORT ANSWER: Answer the following questions (note the points given to each question).

1. Explain why it is important to have a vision for your life. Who is the source of your vision? How do teenagers "borrow trouble?" (10 points)

    With your eyes on a vision (or motivating cause) for your life, the distractions that can hinder you are reduced. Each believer has a purpose for living, a purpose beyond living for yourself. Having a vision for your life.

    God is the source of the vision for your life.

    Teens borrow trouble about: school, friends, etc.

2. What are 5 practical ways that teenagers can be in "hot pursuit" of their destiny in God? (5 points)
    1. *Bible reading.*
    2. *Prayer.*
    3. *Fellowship with other believers.*
    4. *Serving others.*
    5. *Praise and worship.*
    6. *Be aware of the negative influences in life.*

3. Explain the following: "In the same way that a wall is built, stone by stone, you find and walk out your destiny in God a little at a time." (5 points)

    Each brick, when placed in just the right place at the right time, provides extra strength to the structure. As you work to build your life by placing the right principles and commandments together, you will fashion a strong fortress that can withstand opposition. (Luke 16:10, He who is faithful in little, is faithful in much). As you walk out the basic Christian walk, being faithful with what God is doing now, you will find yourself walking in the very purpose God has for your life.

Chapter Sixteen, Test Key, page 2 of 3

4. Seeking a _purpose_ for living means seeking the _creator_ of that purpose. (2 points)
5. Your _goal_ in life is not to decide what _you_ want to do, but to discover what _He_ destined you to do! (3 points)
6. Why is it important not to "borrow trouble?" (5 points)

    It is important not to worry about things that you don't even know will come to pass. Bill Meyer and Dan Zandra say this: We spend so much time thinking about how we might lose, that we forget to think about how we might win. Instead of thinking about how well we're going to do, we spend all our practice time thinking up imaginary disasters for ourselves.

    People need to concentrate on the promises of God. You are on a winning team. There is no way you can lose if you stay on His team. Train yourself, speaking out the promises of God. Be "God-Focused."

7. What are 5 specific disappointments that teens might face and how might these hinder their walk with God? (5 points)

    Any answer would be appropriate (subjective)
    i.e.. family problems, friends

8. What is the meaning of the *cross* in the life of a Christian? (3 points)

    The cross in the life of a Christian is the crossing of two wills, yours and God's.

9. Suffering is saying _"no"_ to _self_ and _"yes"_ to _God._ (4 points)
10. Explain the following verse of scripture. (5 points)

    "And let us not grow weary while doing good, for in due season we shall reap if we do not lose heart." Galatians 6:9

    God knows the struggles you face and that you can become spiritually exhausted from trying to do the "right" thing. You will receive more from God by remaining steadfast.

11. What is the answer to weariness of spirit? (4 points)

    The answer is to wait on the Lord. Wait with patience, anticipation and with humility in His presence.

12. What is your ultimate inheritance in heaven? (4 points)

    To enjoy Jesus Christ forever.

13. How is a person assured of having a place in the Father's house? Does this assurance make your life on earth easier? Why or why not? (10 points)
    Salvation through Jesus Christ as your personal Lord and Saviour.

14. What does it mean to be "God-focused?" Who was an example for us from the Bible? Why is this important in the life of a teenager? (10 points)
    Being "God-focused" is to keep your eyes on Christ even in the most difficult trial. Job was an example for us in the Bible. Through all that he suffered, he endured. He had the kind of loyalty that gave him the power to triumph in the end. Teens go through a lot of emotional and physical changes and challenges. The pressure as a teen to walk away from God is strong. That is why it is so important to stay God-focused.

15. **ESSAY** (25 points) Write an essay entitled:

    "Hindrances to reaching your destiny."

Include in your answer:
- A minimum of 4 hindrances to reaching your destiny. (5 points)
- What is the strongest hindrance? How can a teen overcome this hindrance? (5 points)
- Give a minimum of 1 specific example for each, that may be unique to teens. (5 points)
- Why is it important to have a vision for your life? (5 points)
- Is there a shortcut to reaching your destiny in God? Why or why not? (5 points)

Answer:
  Hindrances:
  - *Lack of motivation.*
  - *Laziness.*
  - *Rebellious attitudes.*
  - *Lack of discipline: learn to discipline the flesh, this being the strongest hindrance to reaching your potential.*

  Vision is a deterrent to sin.
  There is no shortcut to reaching your destiny in God because you must learn from all you go through. There is something in everyone that wants instant results, ultimately avoiding the process of learning. God does not promise that you can avoid or skip over the trials. He does, however, promise to be with you as you walk through them.